CONSULTATION

CONSULTATION
Concepts and Practices

James C. Hansen
State University of New York, Buffalo

Bonna Sue Himes
American Baptist Churches

Scott Meier
State University of New York, Buffalo

Prentice Hall, Englewood Cliffs, New Jersey 07632

Library of Congress Cataloging-in-Publication Data

Hansen, James C.
    Consultation : concepts and practices / James C. Hansen, Bonna Sue
Himes, Scott Meier.
        p.   cm.
    Includes bibliographical references.
    ISBN 0-13-172578-5
    1. Mental health consultation.   I. Himes, Bonna Sue (date).
II. Meier, Scott T. (date).   III. Title.
RA790.95.H367   1990
158—dc20

89-27645
CIP

Editorial/production supervision: Joe O'Donnell
Cover design: Miriam Recio
Manufacturing buyer: Robert Anderson

© 1990 by Prentice-Hall, Inc.
A Division of Simon & Schuster
Englewood Cliffs, New Jersey 07632

Printed in the United States of America

10 9 8 7 6 5 4 3 2 1

ISBN 0-13-172578-5

Prentice-Hall International (UK) Limited, *London*
Prentice-Hall of Australia Pty. Limited, *Sydney*
Prentice-Hall Canada Inc., *Toronto*
Prentice-Hall Hispanoamericana, S.A., *Mexico*
Prentice-Hall of India Private Limited, *New Delhi*
Prentice-Hall of Japan, Inc., *Tokyo*
Simon & Schuster Asia Pte. Ltd., *Singapore*
Editora Prentice-Hall do Brasil, Ltda., *Rio de Janeiro*

CONTENTS

CHAPTER FOUR

CONSULTING IN BUSINESS AND INDUSTRY   118

CHAPTER FIVE

CONSULTATION IN MEDICAL SETTINGS   135

CHAPTER NINE

CONSULTATION THROUGH PROGRAM EVALUATION   220

PREFACE

The age of the consultant has arrived. That there is real need and a market for consultation is manifested by the spiraling requests of school systems, clinics, hospitals, and industry. For instance, industry now employs consultants to assist in screening applicants for positions and to deal with worker-related and interpersonal-systems organizational problems. School systems hire consultants for instructional evaluations, to introduce career education programs, and to deal with interpersonal problems centered around racial or internal staff concerns. Community agencies and hospitals use consultants for program evaluations, organizational development programs, staff development, and case consultations. Individual professionals use consultants for assistance with client diagnosis and treatment planning.

Consultation in mental health and human services refers to a specialized type of helping process wherein an expert or acknowledged specialist endeavors to assist a consultee, which may be a person, group, or system, with some problem related to the consultee's mode of behavior or style of functioning. Consultation is practiced by individuals from a variety of disciplines including psychology, social work, psychiatry, education, and business and management. Mental health consultation differs in two important ways from consultation as it is practiced in other fields. First, it helps to broaden the limited professional manpower that deals with dysfunctional emotional and interpersonal systems problems available to the consultee. Second, it extends the effectiveness of an entire mental health movement so that mental health ideas can have a deeper impact on individuals, community agencies, schools, and businesses.

As with any concept that is in vogue and that has broad ramifications for change in a collective group of professionals, there exists a danger that individuals will embrace new ideas and titles without understanding clearly what the actual shift means in theory and practice. Such is the case with the title of consultant. The consultant is more than a voguish name plate one can use at sheer whimsy. There are concepts and practices that can help the knowledgeable professional to be more skillful in consulting with a person or organization in need.

This book is written as a basic text for individuals preparing to include consultation as part of their professional roles. It will also serve to enhance the knowledge and skills of practitioners who are presently offering consultation services. This book does not present one theory but several major conceptual models. Some consultants adhere to only one model, but most use different models to meet the needs of the presented problem. There is some variation in the procedures and practices of consultation; however, a set of stages in the process is generally followed. This book describes the major concepts and models in the field and an eclectic view of the process, and several chapters are devoted to consultation in specific settings.

The initial chapter discusses many of the concepts in defining what is and is not consultation. Attention is then focused on the various models used to conduct consultation. The final section explores numerous issues or dilemmas that face consultants. This exploration will help readers address the issues in later chapters and think through their ideas before encountering them with consultees. The second chapter presents an eclectic set of procedures and practices that are used in most consultations.

The next three chapters focus on consultation with specific settings. Chapter 3 presents the practices in working with schools; Chapter 4 deals with business and industry; and Chapter 5 applies to medical settings. Chapter 6 presents methods of consulting with groups while Chapter 7 focuses on working with families. Chapter 8 describes the methods used in training and education programs. Evaluation is an important and unique type of consultation and is treated in Chapter 9. The final chapter concentrates on conflict resolution. There are times a consultant negotiates a resolution between two people or groups of people by serving as a third-party consultant.

We are grateful to Harold B. Engen, University of Iowa, and Howard

Splete, Oakland University, Rochester, Michigan, for their reviews of our manuscript.

We have drawn the material in this book from the concepts and research of many writers in diverse fields. We also wish to acknowledge the stimulation of our colleagues and students as an important contribution to the completion of the book. Specifically, we want to recognize Lori Lyth-Frantz, Mark Urich, Lucinda Cornell, Dan Nichols, Mary Maida, and Noelle Berger for their assistance.

CONSULTATION

CHAPTER ONE
CONCEPTS
AND MODELS
OF CONSULTATION

During the last 25 years the development of consultation has been a major addition to the role of mental health professionals. Although they continue to perform traditional activities, consulting has become an increasing aspect of their role, and many have adapted consultation as their primary identity.

Mental health and human service consultants have borrowed concepts and models from the numerous other fields including health, education, business management, and various social sciences. The integration of the knowledge from these fields assists consultants in working with a wide range of consultees and settings.

The role of a mental health consultant is diverse, but most projects involve helping solve problems with individuals, groups, or organizations. The human service aspect of the role focuses on people rather than technology. Organizational consultation involves helping staff solve problems and improve productivity. Both individual and organizational achievement involve complex human interactions, which are the mental health consultant's major focus.

The education of a mental health professional generally provides the background in working with individuals and groups. It takes additional knowledge and experience, however, to function successfully as a consultant. Consultants need to know several models of consultation that will give them alternate ways of looking at problems and different interventions to reach solutions. Consultants also need an understanding of the consultees' organizations, whether they are clinical settings, schools, agencies, hospitals, or businesses. Many of the principles and procedures of consultation will apply across settings, but they need to be familiar with the environment, both technical and social, that will impinge on the consultee and clients.

This chapter discusses several concepts in understanding consultation and then delineates some of the major models in the field of human services consulting. The final section of the chapter examines several important issues that consultants face.

DEFINITION

Consultation is not a new term related to the mental health profession. Under the umbrella of consultation, services can cover a wide variety of tasks. The term has been used to refer to any activity in which an expert provides specialized assistance to another person. In most fields, this means a process in which one professional consults with another. This perspective is differentiated from a treatment situation, with a supervisor and a supervisee, or from teaching, in which the expert is teaching the novice. Human service specialists have modified the concept of consultation to include relationships between professionals in the same field, professionals in different fields (such as a psychologist and a teacher), and also between professionals and lay people such as parents.

Psychiatrist Gerald Caplan (1970) defined *consultation* as

> a process of interactions between two professional persons—the consultant, who is a specialist, and the consultee, who invokes a consultant's help in regard to a current work problem with which he is having some difficulty and which he has decided is in the other's area of specialized competence (p. 19).

Following their review of the literature, Lounsbury and colleagues (1979) appropriately concluded that consultation was a term used to describe a wide variety of activities and relationships. It describes not only the relationship between two professionals working on a case but also the interactions between agencies or professionals connected with them who develop resources, training, or new programs. In general, consultation has been used to describe any meeting between professionals or agencies directed toward improving the quality of service.

Consultation is most often defined by describing what occurs in the process. Bergan (1977) described the activities of consulting as being a problem-solving process. That process begins by trying to obtain a clearer definition of the problem, analyzing the problem, and developing a strategy to solve the problem. Consultation involves a collegial relationship because the consultant and consultee often work as equals in the process. Even when that is not the case, however, the consultant has no authority over the consultee. Consultation involves the utilization of knowledge, and the consultant is sought because of special knowledge and skills. It is through the use of that knowledge that the consultee and consultant are able to develop a solution to the problem. Consultation is often an indirect service. The consultant may not have direct contact with the client, but may work instead with the consultee who provides direct service to the client.

Consultation is triadic in nature, comprised of a consultant, a consultee, and a client. One concept sees the consultee occupying the position between the consultant and client. Thus the consultant works only with the consultee, such as the teacher/parent or the employer, but not with the client, such as the student, child, or employee. The consultant's role is to provide expertise in the problem area and help the consultee work through procedures to resolve the problem. Following the consultation meeting, the consultee then carries out the program with the client. Another concept recognizes that the consultant may work directly with the client as well as the consultee. Thus, the consultant may meet with the student as well as consult with the teacher, or discuss the problem area with an employee as well as meet with the supervisor. This permits the client to contribute to the consultant information that can have an impact on diagnosis and on planning any changes that the consultee will implement in the life situation.

Consultation has also been defined in terms of its relationship with the prevention of mental illness. Parsons and Meyers (1984) describe three types of prevention. Primary prevention is focused on preventing disorder in a population, and the clients may be an entire community or subgroup with mental health problems. Secondary prevention is concerned with problems that are beginning to emerge, with a curative goal, while tertiary prevention provides treatment for the already-present symptoms of dysfunction. The connecting of consultation with prevention developed out of the community mental health movement. MacLean and colleagues (1975) described the consultation process in prevention as consulting with the consultee to assist the management of an individual, family, or family group. It is also concerned with administrations and staffs and their relationships. Consultation helps individuals and agencies to assess the problems of mental health and the need for newer, modified programs. Consultants offer advice on planning, research, training, or service programs as well as evaluation of programs. Consultants teach others about human relations, human growth and development, socializations, and special mental health problems. They also are involved in developing skills in treatment, training, administration, and evaluation, and in the preparation of audio-visual materials.

Consultants carry out a variety of tasks when working with individual consultees or an organization. Gallessich (1982), however, described six common characteristics that generally apply to most consultations: (1) Consultants are experts in specialized bodies of knowledge, and most are experts in the process of helping others solve problems. (2) Consultants work with other individuals and organizations to help them resolve work-related problems, but they only focus on consultees' personal issues as they relate directly to the work situation. (3) Consultation is generally an indirect service in which the consultant serves an agency's clients by working directly with the agency staff. Consultants may meet with clients as a part of the assessment process. (4) Consultants are typically outsiders who develop only a temporary relationship with the consultee or organization. There are times when a consultant is employed in the same agency; however, this greatly modifies the consultant's role and relationships within the organization. (5) Consultation usually occurs between peers whose areas of responsibility and expertise are different. The relationship is voluntary, and each maintains control over his or her involvement. (6) Consultees maintain responsibility for any action eventually taken and are free to accept or reject the consultant's suggestions.

DISTINGUISHING CONSULTATION FROM OTHER ACTIVITIES

There is often a narrow line between consulting and other activities. Consulting is frequently confused with supervising, teaching, and counseling or psychotherapy. Consultation differs from supervision in that supervisors have administrative responsibilities for the outcome and must assure that the work is completed and evaluated. The consultant's responsibility is only advisory; there is no direct responsibility over the consultee.

The consultant offers educational experiences in two ways. The consultant trains through situations that arise out of what the consultee brings to the consultation. Impromptu in nature, training relates directly to the problem at hand. The consultant does not take responsibility for the situation or utilize the formal educational arrangement, but trains instead through the examination of problems. On the other hand, there are times when consultants are hired to provide in-service training for groups of employees or even the general public. Such in-service training may be designed to meet the specific needs of the people attending and uses typical educational methods such as lecturing, audio-visual materials, and role playing.

Consultation also differs from collaboration. Collaborators generally carry joint responsibility. The consultee, by contrast, retains responsibility for the management of the case or program. It may be difficult to distinguish between consultation and collaboration when the consultant is a member of a planning committee or task force that moves from advice giving to the implementation of a proposed plan of action.

There are times when consultation resembles counseling or psychotherapy. This is particularly true when the consultant focuses on the feelings and relationships of consultees. Nevertheless, it is the aim of consultation to be work-related, which sets a clear focus and limitation to the discussion. Although there are times when the personal dynamics of the consultee are involved in resolving work-related situations, consultation is not primarily used for the private motives of the individual consultee.

HISTORY

Gallessich (1982) states that consultation evolved as a result of two social conditions: "(1) existing patterns were no longer adequate to meet crucial societal needs, and (2) knowledge was available that could meet those needs" (p. 17). She goes on to trace the evolution of consultation from ancient prototypes to more recent steps toward specialization.

Consultation has made its greatest gains in the area of mental health and human services in the last 25 years, and has continued to develop in response to human services needs. Interest in this area can be traced to a paper written in 1936 by Lawrence Frank entitled "Society as the Patient." Frank believed that many human problems now lumped together as mental health issues are the outcome of imperfect patterns of social organization. This concept is widely embraced today.

During the 1960s the United States made a new commitment to correcting social ills, and that commitment later influenced the role of consultants. Legislation focused on civil rights issues and services for the handicapped and disadvantaged. One part of this social agenda involved the mental health legislation that provides for services in communities throughout the country. The Mental Health Study Act (Public Law 84-142) led to a nationwide analysis of mental illness. The Joint Commission on Mental Illness and Health (1961) urged more outpatient community mental health clinics, smaller inpatient hospitals, alternative treatment facilities, and mental health education. The commission's message was that more mental health services were needed, that services should be as normalized as possible, and that clients should remain in the community, preferable to institutionalization. The commission also emphasized the need to prevent mental illness through education and consultation within the community. In 1963 President Kennedy signed into law the Community Mental Health Centers Act which made funds available to every state to implement mental health services specifically at the community level. States were divided into "catchment areas" based on population, and federal funds were allocated for construction of facilities and hiring staff. These programs were funded through the division of cost among the community, state, and federal government, with the federal share being the largest. The Community Mental Health Centers Act required centers to provide five essential services: inpatient care, outpatient care, partial hospitalization, emergency services, and consultation and education.

The community mental health movement has had a great impact on consultation. The increased demand for mental health services was so great that consultation was employed as a way of providing greater service to more people. With an insufficient number of trained professionals to staff the inpatient and outpatient centers, programs were established to prepare paraprofessionals. Mental health specialists consulted with other health professionals and paraprofessionals who were providing direct care to the public. The model assumed that if, for example, a mental health specialist consulted with a teacher about a student, not only would the student profit from the new knowledge or skill of the teacher, but the other thirty students in the class would as well. The use of a consultant with other professionals assumed that the knowledge of the consultant would be distributed through them to many other clients.

Following the peak of the community mental health movement came a decline in political support. Cutbacks in federal programs were made, so local communities found it necessary to pursue state funding, and mental health needs competed with other community priorities. Many community mental health facilities have been disbanded or no longer function. With the influence of the community mental health movement, however, the role of the consultant has expanded.

Today, consultation has become a major mental health human service. Consultation is one of the roles of psychiatrists, psychologists, social workers, and counselors. Services are provided to individuals, groups, and a variety of organizations such as hospitals, schools, agencies, businesses, and industries.

MODELS OF CONSULTATION

The concepts surrounding consulting have not reached a sufficiently sophisticated level to be termed theories. The practice of consultation has not evolved from, nor has it been sufficiently systematic and integrated into, general formulations; therefore we talk about models of consultation rather than theories.

The focus and purpose of a consultation may determine the model used by the consultant. The model provides the framework for the interaction between the consultant and the client or consultee. While there are similarities between the models, there are also distinct differences in terms of goals, strategies, and the roles of the participants. In reviewing the following paradigms, these distinctions will become evident. Whether the consultation is designed to provide remediation or education, enhance organizational or individual development, or to prescribe preventive measures, all models involve a problem-solving process aimed at increasing the consultee's effectiveness.

Education and Training Model

When consultation follows an education and training model, it is essentially information oriented with the major function to educate the consultees. The consultant's role is primarily that of an advisor, educator, or trainer, presenting information or training that the consultees can use to better provide service for their agency and clients. The information generally comes from the consultant's area of expertise and, although it may relate to consultee problems, it typically is not focused on resolution of specific problems. This method of consultation permits professionals an opportunity to communicate their expertise to individuals from one or more agencies. It is common practice for agencies to title this form of consultation *staff development* or *in-service training*. The model is consistant with the ideas from the community mental health movement in that one consultant can provide information to a large number of clients (Gallessich, 1982). A later chapter will specially address this approach.

Caplan's Model of Mental Health Consultation

Caplan (1970) is the patriarch of the mental health model of consultation. The consultant uses this model not only to help resolve the problem at hand but to add to the consultee's knowledge or lessen areas of misunderstanding so he or she will be better able to handle future situations more effectively. This is true whether the consultant is working with a single consultee or consulting to a group or a larger organization. Caplan described consultation as a relationship between two professional people and emphasized that their responsibility for the client was left with the consultee. The consultant offers diagnosis, clarification, or advice, which the consultee is able to accept or reject or use in any manner chosen. He believed that consultation is a generic form of specialized professional activity and that mental health consulting is part of the community program for promoting mental health as well as the prevention, treatment, and rehabilitation of mental disorders. Mental health consultation in time became a way for relatively small numbers of professionals to exert an impact on a community through consulting with a large number of consultees, both as individuals and agencies. For a consultee to be truly effective, then, the consultee needed to learn from that consultation and apply those concepts to future situations.

Caplan described the four foci of consultation: on a client, on a consultee, on a program, or on a program administrator.

In the client-centered case, the problems faced by the consultee in dealing with a professional case are the major focus, and the immediate goal is to help the consultee arrive at the most effective treatment for the client. The secondary goal is to increase the knowledge of the consultant, so that he or she may better handle this type of situation with clients in the future. In this model, the consultant's attention is primarily on the client. The consultee will describe the client and the situation to the consultant, and the consultant may meet with the client and use whatever methods of assessment fit his specialization and appear necessary to arrive at an appropriate diagnosis of the nature of the problem. Based on that information, strategies for working with the client are discussed by the consultant and consultee. The consultant pays attention to the consultee's descriptions of the client, reactions to the diagnosis, and possible interventions. By paying attention to the consultee, the consultant will learn about better ways of communicating with the consultee. Too often consultants write reports or verbally communicate only with themselves or someone within their specialization. But when the intervention is to be carried out with the consultee, it is important that the messages from the consultant help the consultee in that process. Although treatment of the client remains the responsibility of the consultee, the responsibility for diagnosis and suggested treatment is the responsibility of the consultant.

As the name suggests, consultee-centered consultation focuses on the consultee. Although it is likely that the problem of a client is the direct reason for the request for consultation—and a successful consultation should lead to improvement in the handling of this case—the consultant's primary interest is to assess the nature of the consultee's work problem and to help resolve it. The consultant spends time talking with the consultee about the client but little or no time talking directly with the client. Consultee-centered consultation occurs, for example, when the consultant finds that a supervisor's attitude or behavior is stimulating an employee into work-problem situations. The consultant understands that because the consultee is having difficulties with the employee, his or her perceptions of the situation are likely to be distorted. In this type of consultation, however, it is the omissions and distortions in the consultee's report about the client that provide the consultant with the basic information. The consultant gains an understanding of the situation by hearing the internal inconsistencies in the consultee's story. When the consultant understands the nature of the consultee's difficulty, he tries to help the consultee resolve the situation through a discussion of the problems of the employee and the supervisor's contribution to their resolution. Being outside the usual consultee–client situation, the consultant brings a certain objectivity that the consultee may be lacking. Through their discussion the consultee may bring to the fore previously overlooked issues and, through this process, gain a better understanding of his or her part in the problem and develop knowledge of him or herself in handling it. Obviously, this approach borders on counseling.

Caplan identified four insufficiencies that interfered with the consultee's ability to adequately handle the mental health problems of a client: lack of understanding of psychological factors; lack of skill or resources in dealing with the problems; lack of professional objectivity; and lack of confidence and self-esteem due to fatigue, illness, or inexperience.

Lack of understanding. In some situations the consultee has not learned the appropriate material to handle the situation with a client. The consultant helps the client by adding to his cognitive knowledge or by clarifying the information about the client so the consultee can see the meaningful interactions within the psychosocial pattern. It is important for the consultant to be aware of the level of the consultee's information so his new information will be consistent with the type and level of knowledge from the consultee's profession. It is important that a mental health consultant not try to turn consultees who are not trained in the mental health field into mental health professionals. This is an expensive kind of in-house training, and it may be more appropriate to use a training program for groups of employees.

Lack of skill. Sometimes the person lacks the professional skill to deal with the complications of the client. The job of the consultant is to assist the consultee in choosing an appropriate plan of action, while insuring that the options which she/he suggests are within the range of actions appropriate to the consultee's level of ability. Obviously, this form of consultation can develop into a situation that is very close to supervision.

Lack of objectivity. Caplan pointed out that even experienced, well-trained consultees occasionally encounter situations in which they are unable to use their skills and knowledge adequately with a particular client. He believes this lack of professional objectivity is due to subjective factors. The consultee's professional empathy for the client or other people in the client's situation may be affected by the consultee's identification or personal involvement, leading to some type of partisanship. In such circumstances the consultee may experience some distortion in judgment, leading to lowered professional effectiveness. Caplan believed there was an interfering "problem theme" intruding into the professional person's functioning. The problem theme is likely to be derived from a longstanding personality difficulty, triggered by something in the client's case or from a current conflict in a consultee's personal life at home or at work. This situation was typically called "theme interference." In such a situation, the consultee usually experiences some degree of emotional upset—ranging from a relatively mild rise in tension to a crisis response—in which general professional functioning and emotional equilibrium are temporarily upset. The consultee is likely to blame his discomfort on problems with the client and displace his feelings of anxiety, hostility, and the like, which the consultant may see as partially originating in the consultee's personal life. The consultant's role in this area is to help separate the person's personal life from the work difficulty and assess the causes of the theme interference. The consultant should focus on finding the nature of the theme in terms of how it affects the work situation. The consultant helps reduce the interference by assisting the consultee in accepting a more reality-based expectation for the client. The consultant deals with the consultee's problems without interfering with the defenses or arousing anxiety and resistance.

Lack of confidence and self-esteem.   When the consultee's functioning is affected by some unspecific lack of confidence or self-esteem, the consultant should apply support. Assuming the consultee is technically competent, the consultant listens to and supports the consultee in a manner that does not weaken the consultee's self-esteem. This type of consultation is more frequently used for professional workers who do not have consistent supervision.

Program-Centered Administrative Consultation

The third type of consultation—centered on the program itself—occurs when a consultee or group of consultees seek assistance with problems in the administration of a program. The problems may relate to planning services or to training effective use of personnel. The consultant's role is to make an assessment of the current program and recommend a plan of action to resolve the difficulties. The consultant frequently involves the consultees in the collection of data about the organization. Because the consultees may have some bias in their reports, the consultant often cross-checks their data with information he has gathered on his own. In addition, through his assessment he can learn about the language and values of the organization so his recommendations for action can be expressed in a more acceptable manner. Consultants generally discuss the information that has been gathered with the consultees. Through these discussions, the consultant will learn their expectations and desires and may help in recommendations for implementation for this particular organization. The consultant may assist in the acceptance of the recommendation by communicating his/her developing ideas in the formative stages so that the consultee group can respond to those recommendations. These can then be modified. Administrative consultants are generally required to present a written report of their assessment of the organization's problems and the recommendations for solutions. Such reports typically deal with short-term solutions of an ideal nature, serving as distant goals toward which an organization may strive.

Consultee-Centered Administrative Consultation

The final type of consultation focuses directly on program administrators. It helps to improve their ability to resolve problems in planning and maintaining their programs and in handling the interpersonal aspects of the operations of their organizations. This type of consultation may involve working with a single administrator or may be applied to a group of administrators in an organization. Although this approach is very similar to the consultee-centered case consultation, it is necessary for the consultant to also have some training in organization and administrative problems. Administrators who opt for this form of consultation are more likely to be open to a psychological or interpersonal approach to administration, since consultation received from the mental health consultant would differ from that received from specialists in their own area.

When working with an individual administrator, the consultant may use many of the same techniques used with "theme interference" in consultee-centered consulting. Again, it is important that his/her role not become one of supervision, nonspecific emotional support, or psychotherapy. Administrative consultation in a group setting is even more complicated. It is best for the consultant to help the group clarify the complexities of a problem; then he contributes to the discussion on the basis of his specialized knowledge of interpersonal motivations and relations. He may help the consultees use group dynamic skills to explore their patterns of interaction in dealing with administrative issues. It is difficult, however, to handle theme interference for the individual in a group situation.

The process.   Mental health consultation involves a process of orderly development. In the early stage, time is spent preparing the group for consultation and establishing the consultation relationship. The process then continues with the assessment of the consultation problem, delivering the consultation message, and ending the consultation and providing a follow-up.

Behavioral Model

Behavioral consultation had its beginnings in the merger of behavioral theory with the practice of consultation. The principles of behavioral psychology lend themselves to a problem-solving approach in consultation appropriate for remediation and prevention. Bergan (1977) is frequently cited as having advanced the behavioral consultation model that remains popular today.

Behavioral psychology has been developed through research and the accumulation of data in both basic and applied investigations. This knowledge base has produced several behavioral principles which proponents offer to explain the "how and why" of behaviors. A fundamental tenet of both behavioral and social learning theory is that problem situations can be understood only in relationship to the environment in which they occur (Bandura, 1969). Both the antecedents and consequences of behaviors are viewed as contributing to any behavioral problem. Thus, there is a concentration on changes in the environment which would either promote a behavior or inhibit the expression of a behavior. A second thesis is that any problem to be dealt with can be stated in an objective and observable manner. A "behavioral analysis" is one step in the behavioral consultation model. These two principles, that behaviors are not the result of client deficiencies but environmental cues and that they can be specified in terms of observable data, guide the behavioral consultation model.

The model assumes that the problems are the result of situational factors (i.e., classroom environment or teacher technique) which can be identified and brought under the control of the consultee in efforts to mediate change. The antecedents to a problem behavior have a wide range and might include behaviors/attitudes of the consultee toward the client, an internal experience of the client, or classroom stimuli, all which may serve to promote the problem behavior. Likewise, consequences can take a number of forms: they can be either punishing or rewarding, or they can be neutral events which can serve to either eliminate or stimulate the behavior.

The focus of intervention and change can occur at either the organizational level or the individual level. In the case of the former, goals might be centered on improving communication (Bergan, 1977; Douglas, 1982; Lennox, Flannagan, and Meyers, 1979) or increasing the ability to problem solve. Consultation in this case would center on facilitating interpretation of information between different groups and on assisting the organization to adopt a decision-making plan, with the use of objectives. The organizational consultation could be problem-specific, for example dealing with racial tension in a system or handling the aftermath of a traumatic event such as student suicide. While the behavioral model lends itself to organizational problem solving, this will not be specifically addressed in the following discussion.

On the individual level, change might focus on remediation or prevention of a particular client's problem, or on consultees' increasing their effectiveness in dealing with problem behaviors. For example, a parent might need help dealing with a child's bed-wetting behavior, and goals might include providing knowledge and techniques to remediate the child's problem. In another case, a teacher might need help dealing with a student's learning disability. Consultation could be provided to the individual teacher or offered as in-service training if it was a typical problem situation. While the behavioral model can be employed in a number of settings, its primary use has been in the area of school consultation.

There are several characteristics of this model. There are two goals of consultation in the behavioral model: (1) to correct problem behaviors of the client and (2) to initiate and maintain consultee behaviors or situational factors which influence the problem behavior of the client (Russell, 1978). This is done in an indirect manner in that the consultant works with the consultee to help her/him to deal with difficult client (or student) behaviors. Rarely does the consultant provide direct service to the client unless modeling is employed in intervention. In addition, this model advocates a collegial relationship between the consultant and consultee. As the consultant generally does not have any authority over the consultee and relies on the professional judgment of the consultee regarding the nature of the problem, equal status in the relationship is necessary. Much of the consultation will take the form of (1) providing education to the consultee as to what situational factors are affecting the problem behavior and (2) communicating how changes might be promoted.

Stages of the Behavioral Model

As outlined by Bergan (1977), behavioral consultation occurs in four stages: problem identification, problem analysis, plan implementation, and problem evaluation. Russell (1978) proposes a five-stage model: observation, functional analysis, objective setting, behavioral intervention, and termination. For purposes of clarity, the following stages will be detailed: problem identification, problem analysis, setting goals and objectives, intervention, and termination. Each stage contains particular tasks which must be completed for successful problem resolution.

Problem identification. We need to determine the behavior to be changed and the desired resultant behaviors. Only by specifying the problem behavior will there be a basis to determine whether there has been a change after intervention occurs. Identifying the target problem behavior can be done by interviewing the consultee or through direct observation of the client or the consultee.

In the interview with the consultee, the consultant will need to ask questions of increasing specificity. Example:

TEACHER: Judy is constantly disrupting the classroom.
CONSULTANT: Tell me some of the things she does when she is being disruptive.
TEACHER: She is constantly out of her seat. She demands attention from other students as well as from me.
CONSULTANT: What is she doing when she is demanding attention?
TEACHER: She will yell to ask for individual help during work periods rather than raising her hand. Or she will go to certain friends for help, interrupting them in their work, if she sees I'm busy with someone else.

In this case, we see that "disruptive behavior" does not provide enough information to determine a particular behavior of Judy's. More specifically, the problem is Judy's out-of-seat behavior and verbal outbursts at a time when what the teacher desires is for Judy to remain in her seat and to ask for help by raising her hand. The question remaining is how many times must Judy be out of her seat to be defined as a problem behavior?

In observing, both the client's behavior and the consultant's behavior are of importance. In the school setting, Goodwin and Coates (1977) cite four student behaviors that need recording (scanning, attending, social interaction, and disrupting) and four teacher behaviors (instructing, rewarding, ignoring, and reprimanding). In addition, variables within the milieu which may interact as other stimuli are noted. The purpose of these observations is to note any relationship between the problem behavior and that of the consultee or the setting (Russell, 1977). This provides information that the consultant can use to determine whether there have been changes in the consultee's behavior or the environment after intervention is initiated.

Problem analysis.   Once a problem has been identified, the next task becomes one of analyzing the behavior. Within this stage, the consultant and consultee attempt to determine what factors might serve to stimulate the problem behavior, what previous attempts the consultee has made to deal with the problem, and what steps need to be taken by the consultee to change environmental cues.

If observation has been employed as the method of determining the problem behavior, then much of the data regarding the problem can be collected for analysis in this prior stage. These data would include the previously mentioned behaviors of both the client and consultee. Of importance are any verbal and nonverbal cues which serve to stimulate the client's problem behavior. These cues may come from the consultee or the environment. Also noted are any consequences that the consultee or environment might impose upon the client in response to the problem behavior.

The client's environment is seen as the primary focus for change and thus the consultant, whose own behavior is a part of this environment, plays an important part. The consultee's actions toward the client are noted, as well as their frequency and the apparent effects on the client's problem behavior. These data are recorded in terms of type, frequency, and apparent relationship between the problem behavior and events from the environment (including consultee's behavior). Other factors might include time of day when the identified problem seems to increase or decrease.

When opting for the consultee interview, these same types of data are necessary to collect for analysis. It also is important for the consultant to explain the principles of behavioral theory which guide this process. The consultee then comes to understand the importance of the environment and can determine what controls might be planned. Once antecedents and consequences of the behaviors have been identified, the task turns to making a plan to modify the environment.

The consultant's role becomes one of asking questions relevant to these connections between the problem behavior and the stimuli which provoke or maintain the behavior. The consultee may be unaware of these connections until these questions are asked and this analysis has been completed. The analysis provides a picture of the interactions from which hypotheses can be made.

The next task is to formulate a plan of action. The consultee, who knows the limitations of the milieu, plays the primary part in formulating a plan. Part of this process may include suggestions from the consultant as to new behaviors which may be required from the consultee. These new behaviors will be required in order to change the pattern and also to maintain any changes that may result on the part of the client's behavior. The consultant must be sensitive to the consultee's ability to carry out any plan formulated. Equally important is the consultee's assessment of the ability to carry out any plan developed.

Setting goals and objectives.   The behavior-change program should be specific. This means determining the objectives of the plan in terms of reducing or eliminating the problem behavior. In the case of Judy's "disruptive behavior," it could mean stating the number of times that Judy's out-of-seat behavior will be tolerated (e.g., two times a day) or eliminated altogether. For example, if the analysis has shown that the teacher has verbally and behaviorally responded (provided a consequence) to Judy's yelling for attention or her-out-of seat behavior, the teacher may wish to try ignoring these behaviors. It may be that the teacher's responses are reinforcing, or are stimulating reoccurrences of the problem behavior. In this case, the plan would specify that when Judy yells for attention, she is ignored. When Judy behaves appropriately by raising her hand the teacher would respond, in an effort to increase the occurrence of this desired behavior.

The purpose in determining specific objectives in terms of desired behavior is to measure the success of the intervention plan. Data, collected throughout the process, provide the clue as to whether the behavior change plan has been successful. It may be necessary to alter the plan if the data do not reflect a reduction or cessation of the problem behavior.

Intervention.   Russell (1978) notes that at times the objectives chosen will require new behaviors on the part of the consultee. The process of collecting the data is in itself a new behavior. To insure that the consultee is able to carry out the goals, it is suggested that the plan be executed in steps. In our example, the teacher would simultaneously be required to stop one pattern of behavior (responding verbally and behaviorally to Judy), while at the same time initiating new behavior (ignoring), while also recording all of these interactions. Russell suggests that it may be more reasonable to implement these new strategies in a gradual manner, so that the consultee can feel comfortable and proficient. This may insure success of the plan chosen since it is less overwhelming. If the plan is too difficult for the consultee to implement, the result will be discouragement of the entire consultation process. Whatever strategies are employed will need to be maintained after the consultation itself has ended.

In order to establish these new behaviors in the consultee, the consultant may be called on to model. This might include modeling how to collect data, how to respond to certain situations, and actual demonstrations to the consultee. The consultant might also employ the behavioral technique of reinforcing the consultee's new behaviors in the intervention through verbal encouragement. If the plan is at all successful and there is an initial reduction of the problem behavior, this will also serve to reinforce the new techniques used by the consultee.

There is always the chance that the consultant will encounter resistance from the consultee. This likelihood can be minimized by reducing the psychological jargon and reducing the burden on the part of the consultee by the active involvement on the part of the consultant (Abidin, 1975).

If the data do not reflect change on the part of the consultee's behavior or the client's problem behavior, then the consultant needs to review the strategy. Determining where changes in the intervention are needed is a joint effort with the consultee.

Termination.   The purpose of the analysis is to determine the frequency of the problem behavior as well as the stimuli which seem to initiate and maintain it. It also provides a baseline from which to measure change after intervention has occurred. Thus the baseline provides an indication as to the success of the strategies used and of the consultation itself. The objectives which have been specified are also used to evaluate the success of the behavior change plan.

If there has been movement towards achieving the objectives, it is likely that the plan selected was effective. It may take time both for the consultee to implement the plan in stages and for the strategies to impact the behavior of the client. Thus the evaluation is in terms of whether the goals and desired behaviors are being attained.

The consultee may continue to need encouragement and praise for the efforts expended in changing her/his behavior. The consultant who recognizes such struggles can help to maintain these behaviors. Encouragement may also help stimulate the consultee to employ the behavior change techniques in other cases of problem behavior encountered.

Even when the primary goals and objectives have been reached, it may be useful to periodically record the initial data to insure that the changes have been maintained over time. The wise consultant will check back with the consultee to determine whether there has been a reoccurrence of the problem behavior and whether the consultation has been successful. Follow-up contacts which have been incorporated into the strategy increase the effectiveness of the consultation services (White and Fine, 1976). Examples of behavior consultation will be used throughout the book.

ORGANIZATIONAL CONSULTING

Whether the consultant is performing individual, small group, or organizational assistance, the opportunity exists to use oneself as a tool for change. This skill is of major importance when doing organizational consultation, as the myriad of possible foci require prioritizing and specificity to guide the direction of the consultation. As with other models of consultation, the purpose of organizational consultation can be aimed at prevention, program development, or problem resolution. The difference is that the purpose or process takes into account an entire system. The process can move vertically and horizontally through an organization; there are many more factors to consider, and required expertise extends beyond the ability to form a helping relationship.

There is much confusion about organizational consultation. Where does one obtain training—in business school, by pursuing a university psychology degree, or in some combination? What does one call such consultants and what are the parameters of their intervention? Do they engage in manager or employee development? Are they trainers and human resource managers, or are they communication and employee relationship specialists (Fitzgerald, 1987)? It appears that organizational consultation runs the gamut, and therein lies a danger; can one consultant hope to develop expertise in such a wide variety of roles?

Organizational consultation lacks a central theory or practice paradigm. There has been relatively little research examining the consultation practice, and implications of various interventions have largely gone unexamined (Fitzgerald, 1987). Lovelady (1984) notes that the work of organizational development (OD) consultants is often based on rudimentary frameworks which do not suggest interventions. "Theory" is often in opposition to reality, and this may be most true for consultation within an organization.

Thus one of the primary tasks for the OD consultant is to engage in a complex diagnosis in which the demands of the organization can be addressed with situationally appropriate interventions. Within these limitations, which might be applied to other models of consultation as well, we shall discuss the peculiarities of organizational consultation as they relate to (1) preentry, (2) initial contact, (3) assessment and diagnosis, (4) intervention, and (5) termination. Primary in the following discussion will be an emphasis on the problem-resolution approach, but other methodologies will be mentioned.

Preentry

Preentry is a time to identify one's values and assumptions about organizations and their relationship to employees. Although theoretically it might be ideal to enter the consultation relationship free of bias, in reality we all have notions about the value and form certain characteristics inherent in organizations might have. These characteristics include the tendencies of organizations to quantify and standardize practices, to use employees for the benefit of a larger purpose (whether for manufacturing of goods or providing social services), and to manage or "control" resources, including employees and material goods.

These characteristics have implications for the consultant in terms of conceptualization of both the "problem" and interventions. Training and experience are of particular importance, since the organization is of obviously great complexity in terms of promoting change and of impact of change over a larger body of both employees and others to whom the organization provides some service. Although the consultant will use many skills common to helping professionals, (i.e., forming a relationship, data gathering, and diagnosis), the OD consultant needs to acquire additional expertise. Entering into OD consultation demands knowledge of systems, hierarchies, and the prevailing mind-sets of managers employing consultants.

Initial Contact

In this consulting model the client is generally a system as opposed to an individual, although not always. At the stage of initial contact, relationship building is the primary task. The consultant and consultee come to an understanding of their particular work styles and the consultee's problem situation.

Change does not come easily.

Certain facts about change often get overlooked in the effort to "sell" the idea that change will produce improved results. Carr (1989) suggests that the process of change includes four common phases. Educating the consultee about these phases is part of the consultant's initial contact.

The first phase of an intervention plan is usually met with excitement, an air of hope and expectation. Yet often there are only vague ideas as to what results will be produced. Following this is a period of hard work as people attempt to implement new procedures and surrender previous methods or habits. Disillusionment can set in and the effort required to carry out change is often questioned. The effort, time, and stress of change are frequently underestimated. Often, an organization will not recognize these factors and how they are related, including their impact on production and morale. The third phase returns to a more hopeful attitude, as new techniques or interventions are seen as having impact. However, there is still increased effort, time, and stress, and the tendency is strong to slip into old modes which require less effort. It is only in the last phase, in which change has been "institutionalized" and effort is now equal to that under previous methods, that change can be seen as successful.

To determine whether consultation is even desired, we might explore whether the need for change is legitimate and who benefits. The realistic demands that will be required need attention (Carr, 1989). In outlining these phases and the considerable time needed for implementation, two objectives are met: the consultee is prepared for the inevitable problems which will occur in the change process, and the style of the consultant is communicated to the consultee. Also provided will be information crucial to the contract formed between the parties, in terms of expectations and a time frame for implementation.

In developing an appreciation for the consultee's workplace, it is suggested that the organizational structure be examined in terms of its culture. Polley (1987) outlines levels which include: myths, symbols, values, goals and norms, objectives, programs, policies, and procedures. By exploring these on an organizational level, we can come to know the assumptions made by management, the specifics that represent these assumptions, and how these are implemented. It also sheds light on any divergent or polarized values of the key players in the organization.

It is suggested by Polley that the myths present in any organization can be reshaped to serve the purposes of change. By proposing certain images, consultants can help organizations develop new myths which can serve to build a new culture for the organization. The consultant who is aware of the current assumptions of an organization will be able to provide images and myths attractive as starting points for change. This concept is useful when organizations are experiencing periods of new development or crisis.

Practical considerations for the organization are also important. What time frame for changes will be acceptable? What are the current potential resources? What are the limitations of these resources, and how will they impact change?

Assessment and Diagnosis

In many ways, assessment begins at the initial encounter. In outlining the change process, the commitment level of the organization can be determined. Other goals of this stage include the continuing collection of data and information, diagnosis, and goal setting.

The problem presented by the consultee will determine the level and type of assessment needed. The consultant's knowledge of systems is crucial, as change in one aspect of the organization will affect the whole. Harrison (1970) proposes that an assessment be made as to level of intervention necessary, for example, at the managerial level or employee level. Intervention is recommended at the level where change will produce enduring solutions, and at the level which can be accommodated within the energy and resources of the organization. The importance of exploring the culture of the consultee's organization is implicit.

An organization is constantly undergoing change. It is not a static entity. Consequently, multiple assessments are necessary and often difficult. The interaction of the organization with external environments, the interaction between internal groups, and the demands placed both internally and externally need consideration. If the organization is a government agency, what are the mandated services? What are the sociopolitical implications for change on both employees, management, and citizens? What are the budget constraints or grant possibilities?

In the case of a corporation, what is the attitude toward management? What is the leadership style? Is management participatory or not? What are the market demands, and how will a probable initial reduction in productivity (as new methods are learned and implemented) affect the company?

In some respects, diagnosis must be multidisciplinary. Looking at organizational environment, the historical patterns, the functional patterns, the adaptability of the organization for change, the future growth and goals, the political climate, and the personalities of the participants require distinctive competencies (Hirschowitz, 1978).

One diagnostic process (Kelner, 1984) examines the current situation, causes of the situation, and direction of change. In looking at the current situation or problem, all parties exchange their perspectives on the facts, meanings, and implications. Next, strengths and deficits are noted as contributors to the situation and, finally, a decision is made as to what methods of evaluation and goals will be utilized. Kelner outlines a four-step sequence: exploring perspectives, organizing diagnostic perceptions into a framework, identifying problems and goals with the consultee, and prioritizing goals.

Although there might be pressure to start problem resolution immediately, coming to a consensus as to the definition of the problem and its likely causes will be time well spent. In the first step of exploring perspectives, the consultant's own view and contributions can be important. Often an outsider can express an outlook that an "insider" fears to express or cannot see due to lack of objectivity. In organizing the information shared in the first step, it is suggested that three core areas be addressed: personnel, programs, and the system. Data should be categorized as either perceived strengths or deficits in these three areas, with all parties providing input. Feedback to all parties provides the opportunity for clarification of perceptions and problems. This leads to the opportunity for goal setting, with the next step to prioritize those goals. In prioritizing, the questions are: Where are we now? Where do we want to be? How will we get there? (Lovelady, 1984.)

The most important aspect of assessment and diagnosis is to provide feedback to all parties involved. In the process of gathering data, assumptions can be questioned and new perspectives developed. Techniques such as brainstorming, surveys, and questionnaires can be developed to provide information in this process. This is not a simple procedure. Feedback may generate additional concerns, ideas, and priorities. There is much overlap between this stage and the others.

It is easy to become overwhelmed with the process of assessment and diagnosis. Because of the numerous types of organizations to whom consultants are called upon to provide OD expertise, and the infinite number of problem situations which might be presented, guidelines for assessment are often cursory. There are, however, some general rules of thumb that are helpful. First, involve the organizational players who will be required to implement any interventions. Their investment in the process of problem identification will help carry them over the "hump" when motivation starts to wane under the stress and effort that change will require. Second, recognize that resistance is inherent in change because it requires loss of previously valued "assets"—attitudes, habits, methods, techniques—which may have "worked" at one time. Finally, realize that managers often deal in the objective and concrete world of numbers, budgets, and personnel productivity. Appreciate this perspective while also keeping the more abstract issues of motivation, planning, and problem solving in focus. Helping the consultee understand these issues as they relate to his "everyday" work situation will facilitate communication.

Intervention

At the intervention stage the consultant will confront excitement, hope, energy, resistance, fear, and possible sabotage of change efforts. It is the stage during which employees have the opportunity to implement their new training with optimism regarding improved outcomes. But inadequate preparation for change, without input from all concerned parties, can also contribute to resistance to change. Fears about the outcomes, acknowledgement of frustration, increased work time and demands on concentration, and stress on the parties affected need to be addressed.

There are six organizational interventions (Kurpius, 1985) which the OD consultant may employ: (1) Human resource development includes interventions aimed at increasing human productivity or that are directed at increasing human potential and resources. (2) Survey feedback/action research is a diagnostic intervention. It seeks to gather information about an entire system for the purpose of selecting specific and appropriate interventions. Surveys are typically employed to obtain data used to identify problems and improve the functioning of the organization. (3) Organizational culture building is used to examine the myths and assumptions of the workplace, its patterns of interaction and its climate. (4) Strategic planning and choice-making involve planning for the future. Creativity and risk taking are encouraged in attempts to make the organization proactive rather than reactive to the environment. (5) Job design/enrichment focuses on improving the quality of life in the work environment by redesigning job tasks in some manner. It is an attempt to influence an employee's behavior, motivation, and satisfaction by examining skills, task significance, and meaningfulness. (6) Management by objective (MBO) involves setting specific obectives in order to define organizational goals and increase motivation. Implied is that workers have needs for achievement which will best be met by individual goal setting. With support by managment for this individual appoach, the employee will have greater motivation. However, for organizational maintenance, these individual objectives must be both rewarded and linked to the larger organizational objective.

These different objectives for the consultation will naturally involve various and multiple intervention strategies. Other aspects of the consultant's role during this stage are provided by Lovelady (1984). Besides the general client-centered consulting, the following activities may be required: training and development, liaison and dissemination, counseling, and self-development. These categories were determined by consultants in the field who felt called upon to offer these services to employing organizations. Planning, problem solving, learning, process consultation, and structural change all involve differing degrees of these interventions.

In this research (Lovelady, 1984), consultants were unable to provide concise reasons for implementation of one type of intervention over another, but it was noted from their descriptions that they fell into five basic considerations. One is the skill of the consultant and his/her prior experiences with as particular intervention (e.g., questionnaires). The second is the perceived expectation of the consultee in terms of what would occur. A third selection factor is cost, in terms of money and resources. The level of intervention and the type of data available, as well as the culture and norms of the organization, were the last two aspects affecting the intervention chosen. It was noted that unstructured techniques were generally avoided as it was perceived that management would not tolerate them.

In summary, the intervention strategies planned required that the consultants balance their own skills and knowledge with the needs, desires, expectancies, and norms of the consultee's organization. This means that interventions are complex and require that individual situations be taken into account. Consultants may need to take a more active role in this model, both for diagnosing and planning interventions. They are "doers" as well as helpers.

Termination

The time for termination can be determined by either the consultant or the organization. This decision may occur prior to actual implementation of the intervention plan. Much of the time the impact of intervention strategies are long term, thus evaluation is difficult and determining the success of one intervention over another often impossible to calculate. Consultation with an organization is dependent upon the support given to the process, the time frames used to implement changes, future demands placed on the organization, and the skills of the consultant. The power of the consultation is related to the distribution of power in the organization, whether it be in terms of leadership or collective-bargaining issues. Thus, evaluation, generally occurring in this stage, may be a long-term process. Much depends on the original focus for change, whether it is systemic in nature or a training component.

The advantage of this model is that organizational training, structural change, and future planning can have long-term beneficial effects. This model can promote continuous examination of various organizational tasks, procedures, and norms which are missing in less-comprehensive models.

The Process Model

Schein (1969) presented the "process model" as a practical description of how the consultant works in an organizational development consultation. Although written about organizational consulting, the concepts are as useful in working with individuals and groups. As a preliminary to presenting his model, he described two other models and their weaknesses. It is worth reviewing those models to see the misconceptions that can interfere with successful consultation.

Purchase model.   Schein (1969) described the most prevalent model of consultation as the "purchase model" since the consultee asks for or "purchases" the expert's knowledge or service. The "buyers" or consultees define something they want to know or have done which they or their agency cannot do, and a consultant is hired to provide it. Schein notes that consultees frequently express dissatisfaction about the consultation they receive. Such comments are understandable, however, when all the variables involved in successful consultation are considered. First, the consultee must have correctly diagnosed his/her own needs. Consultees frequently do not know specifically what they need, knowing only that there is a problem. If a consultant does what is asked but does not meet the specific need of the consultee or that organization, it will lead to an evaluation of ineffectiveness. Success is also dependent on the consultee's ability to correctly communicate those needs to the consultant. Again, if the consultant accepts at face value what is asked, he may not meet the actual needs of the consultee. Success with the purchase model also requires that the consultee accurately assess the consultant's ability to provide the right service. If the consultee hires a consultant who does not have the specific expertise, the consultation will likely be ineffective. A fourth requirement involves the consultee understanding the consequences of having a consultant do the job. If he has not examined the consequences of implementing the consultant's recommended changes, he may only discard the report or only change what the consultant has helped to implement.

Doctor–patient model. Another popular model of consultation described by Schein is the "doctor–patient model." This model is frequently used when providing an evaluation of a program. The object is to have the consultant evaluate a program, determine what is wrong or could be improved, and then recommend strategies to establish the improvement. Many members of the consultee's organization, however, may be reluctant to reveal these kinds of information. Individuals worried about job security may hide information, which interferes with an accurate diagnosis. On the other hand, some individuals use the consultation interview as a gripe session and exaggerate the problems in areas of dissatisfaction. Thus it may be difficult for the consultant to gain an accurate assessment of the consultee system. Another problem arises when the consultee is unwilling to believe the diagnosis or accept the consultant's recommendations. Many consultant's evaluations are merely placed in a file. A different difficulty of the doctor–patient model occurs when the consultant does the evaluation and then leaves. The consultee system may have problems implementing the recommendations. Consultations are often considered to be ineffective only because the consultee organization does not have the expertise to implement a recommended plan.

The process model. Schein describes the "process model" as a set of procedures that are likely to lead to success. Because a consultee often does not know exactly what the problem is, the consultant needs to involve the consultee in the diagnostic process. The cooperative diagnostic process will not only lead to a clearer statement of the problem but, more importantly, to the acceptance of the needed interventions. The consultee may also not know the kinds of help the consultant can provide, so one of the early consulting tasks is to determine if the consultant can provide the right expertise. If not, the consultant can help the consultee find the right person. This model places emphasis on the fact that consultees have a constructive intent to improve things and that, when given help in identifying the problems and carrying out the recommendation, success is likely. Consultees can be effective when they learn to diagnose their own strengths and weaknesses. Consultants need to have a joint working relationship with consultees, who really know the situation, and learn enough about the client system to make good recommendations. Following a shared diagnosis, the consultee can be active in generating remedies and implementing the interventions.

Schein (1978) described the process-consultation model as really having two versions: the catalyst model and the facilitator model. The catalyst model occurs when the consultant does not know the solution but has skills in helping the client establish his own solution. The facilitator model is used when the consultant has ideas of possible solutions but decides that a better solution or better implementation of that solution will occur by helping the consultee to solve the problem.

The consultant's major role is to provide new alternatives for the consultee to consider. The decision of what to do always remains with the consultee. This model puts emphasis on the consultant being an expert in the diagnostic process and establishing working relationships with the consultee. Actually, interpersonal process skills form the major area of expertise. Even so, it is important to have expert knowledge in the areas which need attention.

A META-THEORY

Gallessich (1985) described the practice of consultation as generally atheoretical and intuitive. Although several models of consultation have been developed, theory and research lag far behind practice. To overcome this problem, she proposed a consultation meta-theory. She intended to unify the scattered and heterogeneous concepts by identifying their fundamental similarities and differences, and to present a guide to practice, research, and training in the field of consultation.

In developing her paradigm, she identified five parameters common to all approaches to consultation. First, all consultation has content through the body of knowledge consisting of the concepts, principles, and techniques of the consultant. Second, although they vary from task to task, all consultation approaches have goals. Third, all models of consultation have rules for the roles and relationships between the consultant and consultee. Generally the relationship is described as one in which both members volunteer and in which the consultee retains responsibility and authority for the final decisions. Fourth, all models involve a set of processes through which the consultant works to achieve the goals of the situation. Fifth, all consultation models are based on ideologies or value systems which are determined by the consultant. Although not clearly described, the consultant's ideologies and values affect the goals and other variables of the consultation process.

Following the five common parameters in previous models, Gallessich proposed three new configurations. The differences in these approaches to consultation are found in their value systems or ideologies.

The scientific–technological model is founded on the belief in the scientific method. Problems are seen as knowledge deficits, and the goal is to provide appropriate information. The consultant's role is to provide technological expertise, and goals are achieved by using cognitive processes in applying the knowledge and techniques.

The human-development model is logically concerned with human growth and development, and problems are seen as the consultee's personal and professional developmental needs. There are two assumptions in this approach which lead to different roles and procedures. Using the therapeutic approach, the consultant takes responsibility for the assessment and intervention to enhance the development of both the consultee and client system. Using a collaborative approach, the consultant and consultee assess the problem and evolve interventions together. The consultant's role is primarily educational and facilitative with both approaches, and includes both affective and cognitive processes.

The social–political consultation model is concerned with the political or social perspective of the consultee's work and organization. Problems are seen from partisan perspectives. The goal is to change organizations to make them more consistent with particular values, and the consultant is to assume a partisan position.

Conclusion

These major models for consultation will be more clearly delineated in the following chapters. Chapter 2 will describe a generic set of stages in the process of consultation. The stages do not follow a specific model but form an eclectic model of the process. The remaining chapters will focus on a particular type of consultation, and various models will be used as examples.

ISSUES CONSULTANTS FACE

Consultants will confront numerous issues which affect their mode of behavior, acceptance, and eventual success. For the purposes of this discussion we have defined an issue as having at least two sides without a definitive answer—if there was, it would not be an issue. An issue exists when there are different possibilities, different ways of behaving that affect the outcome. The purpose of this discussion is to present some of the issues which consultants may face. Exploring issues before they arise and anticipating the consequences of alternative decisions may lead to more effective resolutions. Examining some issues at this point in the book may also improve understanding of issues presented in later chapters.

Type of Organization

Whether the consultant is working with an individual within an organization or the total organization, an awareness of the differences that exist between private, public, and third-sector organizations has some impact on the consultant's work style.

Consultation in the private sector involves dealing with the philosophy behind task-oriented and profit-motivated organizations. Organizational concerns are typically related to products and more impersonal factors, such as materials, machinery, plants, offices, which are involved in producing the goods and services that the organization provides. When human services or mental health consultants are engaged with this type of organization, they are usually focused on helping employees reduce stress or some other personal variable which will eventually lead to a more effective and more productive employee. Many organizations from this perspective are not only concerned with the money spent in hiring the consultants but in the money lost in terms of employee time spent with the consultant rather than working.

Consultation in the public sector involves working with the federal, state, and local organizations. These may include health departments, school systems, and correctional institutions. Most of these organizations are bureaucratic in structure. Typically, these organizations have few or no competitors, and the absence of competition may leave the system more complacent about itself and the services it offers. However, at the same time, public sector organizations are subject to diverse pressures at many levels. Consultants need to have an awareness of the patterns and behaviors that tend to typify public agencies. For example, administrators tend to maximize information and control at the upper levels of the organization and may be reluctant to delegate authority. There tend to be legal specifications regarding appropriate and inappropriate work behaviors and a strong need for security. Public agencies also tend to stress procedural regularity. Likewise, the concept of the professional manager is less well established in the public sector than in the private. A consultant's understanding of the differences that occur between the public and private sector and the awareness that these are naturally occuring phenomena will help understand the process that occurs during the consultation. For example, these differences may have an impact on the range of changes that can be considered as well as impact on the timetable for the creation of change.

Third-sector agencies are neither public nor private and often are nonprofit. They tend to be service deliverers rather than producers of products. These organizations, often characterized by a concern with the redress of social inequities, have roles as agents of social change. Third-sector agencies tend to have general directions or interests leading to ambiguous and often incompatible and contradictory goals. The management system may be highly flexible in order to achieve more social responsiveness. Therefore, there are times that decision making is accomplished not by making a decision but by letting it emerge. Although the range of third-sector agencies is large, these institutions tend to be more flexible, innovative, independent, and probably more problematic than other forms of institutions. The differences between private, public, and third-sector institutions will become apparent to the consultant working in these three types of organizations.

Consultation and Role Confusion

In many human-services consulting situations a primary issue is to differentiate between consulting and counseling with the consultee. There are also times when consultation and supervision may be intertwined and/or confused. The issue of differentiating consulting and counseling occurs most frequently when there is a consultee-centered consultation in process. Does the consultant counsel with the consultee, in an effort to facilitate understanding and a comprehension of the consultee's relationship with the client, or is the focus only external, on the client? At times the consultant may focus on the consultee's feelings, attitudes, and values regarding a particular client. Under such circumstances the line between counseling and consulting is not always clearly drawn. Even though it is important to help the consultee understand him or herself in terms of the job with the client, the ultimate objective of helping the client can be neglected or avoided entirely. Consultation is a process that focuses on the external or the client's problems, and therapy with the consultee should be avoided.

It is not uncommon for the consultee to feel more comfortable after the consulting relationship has been established and the two people come to know each other. At these times the consultee may explore issues in his personal life which are similar to the work situation. Teachers may talk about their children at home, describing situations not dissimilar from what happens in their classrooms. Managers may also talk of situations in their private lives.

There are two approaches the consultant can use when this occurs. One is to listen to the consultee and then refer them to someone else to focus directly on their personal problem, if that is what they are interested in. Another approach, when it is appropriate, is for the consultant to suggest to the consultee that their discussion is now moving towards counseling and away from consulting. If the consultee wishes to continue in that kind of relationship, it needs to be part of their verbal contract, so both know what they are involved with. The issue of the consultant functioning both as a consultant and a counselor obviously poses additional problems, including the ethical issue of a dual relationship. In a counseling situation the counselor is in control of the process from an expert position. By contrast, the consultant controls the process but has no real power. The consultant and consultee function more as equals of different specialization. They have a professional, collegial relationship.

Particularly after an intervention has been agreed upon and the consultee has implemented it, the consultant could be moved into a position of supervision. It is important to make clear the differences both in responsibility in the roles as well as in power and control. A supervisor is responsible to the agency to insure that the performance of the employee meets standards and expectations, whereas the consultant has no responsibility for the consultee's quality of performance. A supervisor has expectations and administrative authority over the supervisee, which establishes a superior–subordinate relationship. The consultant has no authority in establishing standards of performance, and the consultee is not held accountable for following through. The relationship becomes much different and can lead to serious problems on the job when the consultant functions as a supervisor.

Expert or Collaborator?

Another issue centers around the involvement by the consultant throughout the consulting process. This specific issue concerns active versus passive participation by the consultant. The consultant may assume a role of very active participation in the consultation, searching for solutions to the problems and making recommendations largely on his or her own. Such a position is often described as the expert model. The consultee may be relied on for varying degrees of feedback, but decisions are made primarily on the expertise of the consultant. The recommendations, however, must ultimately be implemented by the consultee and, therefore, the consultee should work toward developing a trusting relationship with that person. This suggests some degree of involvement by the consultee, but he or she definitely remains the secondary partner when the consultant works as an expert. The other point of view holds that the greatest responsibility must ultimately be placed on the consultee for seeking solutions to problems. It emphasizes the establishment of a close working relationship between the parties, which hopefully will lead to both sharing equally in the solution to the problem at hand.

According to Martin and Meyers (1980) the attribution of expertise to consultants is positively related to a positive consultation outcome. Clearly when we ask a person for his or her advice we want to talk with someone whom we consider to be more knowledgeable and experienced than ourselves. To consider certain people as experts is to hold a comfortable belief, especially when we need answers. The term "expertise" refers to the belief that the consultant is an expert problem solver. When this belief is carried to extremes, however, consultees may take a passive approach to a problem, assuming that the consultant can handle the problem better and therefore should be allowed to do it. For example, Dinkemeyer (1984) reported that some teachers believe the school counselor should "fix" problem children. Some teachers believe that problems with certain students are not their responsibility and may go so far as demanding that the counselor directly confront the problem at hand. Yet, the teacher works with the student everyday and has a greater potential impact on the student. Also, if the consultant excludes teachers, they may eliminate ways of changing the teachers' attitudes about the student in question, which would also have an impact on the outcome.

Steele (1969) concluded that consultation should involve three major factors: (1) the levels of expertise should be balanced, (2) the entire responsibility for decisions should not be placed in the hands of the consultant, and (3) all forms of expertise should be shared.

Educational professionals prefer collaboration over more indirect service models (Babcock and Pryzwansky, 1983). Babcock and Pryzwanski point out that it does not necessarily follow that because the consultee prefers a certain approach, that approach is the most effective one. Some variables have been identified that affect teacher cooperation. The same variables fit with most other consultees. The variables include the amount of effort required, the consultant follow-up, and whether interventions are designed in ways that are congruent with the teacher's perception of his or her role (Sattler, 1982).

The consultant is often viewed by the consultee as an expert. He or she may be expected to pass along relevant information and knowledge to the person of lesser expertise. While such a perception may benefit the consultant by increasing the likelihood that he or she may be listened to, it also negates the strength of the consultee and ignores the need of the consultant for assistance in the diagnostic process. To achieve the best resolution to the consultee's problem the consultant must work in collaboration with the consultee.

Among costs to the consultee when he or she becomes too heavily dependent on the expert is that the consultee may become overly dependent on the consultant and fail to develop his or her own diagnostic problem-solving skills. As a result the consultation would yield only short-term gains.

Emphasis on the consultant as an expert may lead to inadequate solutions. Better choices in courses of action are likely to be found when the consultee's past knowledge of the situation is combined with the consultant's area of expertise. While the amount of collaboration between the consultee and the consultant may vary, it appears that a joint effort to find solutions is optimal.

Accountability may be a closely related aspect in this issue. How responsible should the consultant be for implementing change as a result of the consultation? One point of view suggests that the consultee has the power to "take it or leave it" in terms of making use of the consultant's recommendations. At the opposite viewpoint, the consultant is to be a motivator of action and should seek powerful figures to back his recommendations.

The consultant is responsible for looking for accountability for his or her work. If the consultation is not perceived as successful, is it because of a wrong solution, or has the consultee not carried through due to lack of ability or not being willing to make the changes?

Gaupp (1966) differentiated between authoritative and authoritarian elements in consultation. The authoritative component involves the power elements that are based on knowledge while the authoritarian elements include the aspect of enforcement. Gaupp suggested that in moving toward freedom in decision making, the consultant's role should be decreasingly authoritarian and increasingly authoritative.

Follow-Through

A further issue regarding degree of involvement concerns duration and process. Does the consultant move on quickly in working through possible courses of action, or does he/she continue his/her participation through the implementation stage and assist in the evaluation of the courses of action? A temporary consultation may provide feasible solutions to a problem, but the ideas may provide only short-term relief. A briefer consultation could lack depth of involvement and may result in the lesser ability to understand the intricacies of the consultee's problems and the reluctance of the consultee to divulge important information. Although Steele (1969) favors a temporary involvement, he notes that such involvement may serve as a flight from a necessary deeper involvement in a particular problem, that is, working it through, and this may reduce the client's willingness to provide important data or impair the consultant's ability to understand the situation. He also points out that working on several cases at the same time can lead to conflicts in amount of time and energy available and emotional commitment.

There are times that agencies have sufficiently complicated problems that only an ongoing consultation can provide an adequate resolution to the problems. Nearly all consultants believe their duties involve working through problems with the consultee, including a joint evaluation of the new procedures that have been implemented. An ongoing consultant may become more of a staff member. In that situation she/he is still part-time and, therefore, in a marginal position. Other employees may not view the consultant as a full-fledged staff member, and the consultant, too, may feel the same. This lack of role clarification within the agency may reduce role acceptance as well. Although serving as a continuing consultant is frequently a problem, it is not without advantages. Such a consultant may possess several of the strengths listed for the internal consultant, therefore increasing his overall effectiveness. And the marginal nature of the position may help the person avoid the assumption of other staff responsibilities and policy-making functions.

Inside or Outside the Organization?

Is it possible for a person to function as a consultant inside a school, business, or agency when he or she is a member of the staff? Or is the consultation more effective when the person is outside the system? Can someone who is part of the organization, and possibly part of the problem, be sufficiently objective to serve as a consultant? Would it be better to bring in an objective person from the outside who is less involved with the consultees?

When consultees ask for help from an outside consultant, it is obvious they feel that the existing resources within the organization, whether a school, hospital, or clinic, cannot solve the problem. Many organizations have now employed internal assistants such as management analysts, development specialists, and industrial psychologists, and some part-time employees function to assist in staff relationships.

There are some advantages for the inside consultant including closer communication links, richer interpersonal relationships, and the possibility of trust and respect. There are times when the internal consultant has the advantage of added insight into the source of the problem and knowledge of how the organization works.

An inside consultant has the advantage of familiarity of the structure of the organization, both the formal and informal networks and power bases of individuals. An outside consultant may not recognize some important hidden agendas and may miss subtle alliances which need to be addressed for successful resolution of the problem.

An inside consultant may be perceived as having more vested interest in the need to solve a particular problem and may get more support from the consultees or clients. The consultant may be seen as "one of us" and therefore someone to work with rather than against. The outside consultant may be seen as not really recognizing "what it's really like" since he/she has not been in the organization. The advice may be discounted as unrealistic and unworkable without receiving fair consideration. It is important for a consultant working within the system to create an image that reflects his concern for the clients rather than one that appears to be supervisory or management oriented. To deal with this situation the internal consultant needs to be willing to test the degree of freedom he has and possibly increase it. Because the inside consultant is part of the organization, his freedom to operate may be restricted and, therefore, the situation must be tested.

The external consultant often is perceived with more credibility because the perceptions are considered objective and shaded by personal involvement in the organization. The external consultant also has the ability to maintain a detachment from the client's problem that can be uniquely helpful to the client. Although a person functioning as an internal consultant may have experienced the atmosphere of the system and have a firsthand knowledge of the perceived problems, this person may be blinded by these details.

The internal consultant may be affected by the problem situation and may tend to act in his or her own best interests. Knowing the other personnel involved at a more personal level, opinions and impressions have already been formed that may lead the consultant to consider more factors than is necessary for the problem under consideration. An internal consultant needs to maintain constant vigilance regarding personal needs versus professional responsibility. The consultant must interact with the consultee as well as the client. The consultee and clients have also formed previous impressions of the consultant which may increase their resistance. If the consultant has an established role in the mind of the consultees, it might be an additional barrier to overcome, or it could be an advantage to already have that level of acceptance.

Nufrio (1983) mentioned problems of collecting data that can arise from working within an organization. The consultee might hold back information from the very people who are trying to help, thereby frustrating efforts to collect data necessary for problem analysis and resolution. Nufrio implied that such "information isolation" might come about because the consultant was closely associated with the administration. The other side of this situation can occur when the inside consultant becomes too closely associated with the consultee organization and its problems and may overidentify with the consultees, thereby losing objectivity.

By a consultant being an external agent, a higher degree of objectivity may be possible due to the freedom from restraints and from personal gain or loss. The consultant should have no administrative responsibility over the consultee's work or job security and vice versa. When the consultee is an administrator in the organization who can have the consultant fired, the internal consultant may think twice regarding some honest assessments.

Another concern is a consultant's degree of accountability to the organization. An internal consultant is often considered more accountable and responsible to the organization. Given greater accountability, however, the internal consultant may be less willing to risk organizational changes. While an internal consultant may be concerned with the burdens of responsibility and accountability, the external consultant should be cautious in this regard.

Gluckstern and Packard (1977) summarize the advantages and disadvantages inherent in being an inside or outside consultant. The advantages to being an inside consultant include having familiarity with the structure of the organization, its goals, channels of communication, and how it functions. It is easier to talk with peers and find out sources of valid information that help in data gathering. The person also has a better understanding of the politics of the organization. The disadvantages of an inside consultant include being taken for granted by his/her peers. Often the setting is not as formal and structured as it should be and therefore the consultations may appear slipshod in manner. The informal initiation of the process may undermine the professionalism of the consultant. The insider may become enmeshed—that is, it is difficult to remain objective—or may even become controlled by the setting because of job security. The insider may have difficulty taking a position which alienates peers, and often an insider's recommendations are less likely to be taken seriously by peers.

The outside consultant has the advantage of being more impartial and less constrained by peer pressures. The external consultant can play an advisory role and not have to be involved in the implementation of the plan. These consultants usually do not have administrative control over the consultee, but bring in information and experiences from a broader resource base. The external person has an ascribed status and is credited with special knowledge and given special sanctions. It is especially easier for a consultant from outside the organization to work with administration-centered consultation. The primary disadvantage for the outside consultant is the increased effort required to become familiarized with the organization and to understand the intricacies that an inside person would know well.

Confidentiality

Confidentiality is an issue that requires considerable attention. One position holds that confidentiality is not a part of the consultation process in that all information that increases the possibility of aiding the client should be shared by the consultant and consultee. For example, if the consultant is working with a manager on problems which the manager has with one of the employees, the consultant, as well as the manager, should be entirely open in presenting all information that is pertinent to the situation. If the consultant does not share pertinent information, the consultee may feel slighted. Lack of information may interfere with the consultee effectively diagnosing and or resolving the situation.

On the other side of this issue, it is suggested that much of the information between the consultant and client is confidential and should not be shared with anyone unless the client agrees to such a disclosure. If employees in organizations, students in school, or staff in an agency believe that what they tell the consultant is not held in confidence, they will not participate in data gathering or disclose information necessary for consultation to be successful. The discussion of supposedly confidential information with others will result in loss of the consultant's credibility with the client, sometimes with other clients, and possibly even with the consultee. This may be one of the most difficult issues to resolve.

There are times when a consultant is caught between obligations to the consultee, client, and the organization. For example, the consultant reassures that the consultation will be constructive and helpful to the consultee, while at the same time being protective of the needs and rights of the client. Obligations to the client may be in conflict with the organization's obligations to other members. Should decisions be based on the well-being of the individual or of the organization? It is important that the consultant recognize the situation before it becomes too complicated so it can be discussed with the consultee. It is also appropriate for the consultant to discuss with the consultee and client what types of information will be shared, so that each is aware of what type of material will be held in confidence and what will not.

Yeager (1982) listed confidentiality as the issue having the greatest impact on consultation. The consultant is responsible for both facilitating human relations and meeting business priorities. When the consultant is working with an organization, the funding is usually covered by that organization. When a consultant is working in an organization to improve some area of weakness, the process probably involves some evaluation of specific departments or individuals. When the evaluation is completed, the consultant has the responsibility to help change areas of weakness in the organization. Yeager believes that a consultant should "encourage clients to reveal necessary data (i.e., results of the evaluation) to their supervisors" (p. 598). If the clients reveal the important data regarding themselves and their programs it removes the consultant from concerns regarding confidentiality. If the clients are not involved in that process and the consultant makes the report, he or she is responsible to communicate important information without breaking individual confidentialities. Hengeveld and Rooymans (1983) report a study of 313 consultants in a hospital setting that seemed to support Yeager's position when they concluded that a more open postevaluation approach helped to alleviate a major obstacle in the consultation's success.

Resistance

One of the key issues in the consultation process involves the consultee's and possibly client's resistances to the process and the consultant's ability to involve them in it. Some consultee resistances are seen as coping devices, such as unrealistic expectations; misconception of the purpose of the consultation; testing out the consultant's investment, conviction, and ability to help them; evading the consultation by means of scapegoating, self-blaming, or open resistance.

Resistances frequently occur during the assessment and diagnosing stage. Fears and anxieties regarding diagnosis surface in a number of ways, and a consultant needs to recognize various forms. One frequent behavior involves checking the consultant's credentials. A consultee may ask, "Have you ever worked in a healthcare or community agency before?" While these are legitimate questions, the consultant needs to be aware that they may arise from resistance and anxiety. Departments of an organization into which the consultant is moving may perceive the consultant as a threat. They may feel it is due to their failures that the consultant has been brought into the organization. Under such circumstances individuals may not disclose or may even distort certain information in the data-gathering process.

The concern regarding confidentiality is legitimate and sometimes raises resistance. If a client provides negative data about the organization, will he or she be identified in a manner that could have negative consequences? The consultant needs to provide appropriate reassurances, but this anxiety can also represent a further instance of resistance.

Consultants recognize that everyone is apprehensive about change. People become adaptive to the present situation although they may complain about it. Any change may be in directions that are less advantageous, and thus they will approach them with ambivalence. A consultant needs to recognize and provide a period of testing in which the resistance and ambivalence about his or her role will be a major concern of some consultees and clients.

Professional knowledge and self-confidence are needed when the consultant's recommendations are not readily acceptable or attainable. The consultant needs to accept the feelings of the consultees and clients and use the process to help them become involved in working through to an agreeable resolution. This begins by recognizing such messages as coping devices and communicating to staff that it is appropriate to ask such questions and raise such issues. In fact, helping consultees with their concerns and problems becomes part of the consultation process. If the consultant involves consultees and clients, they are more likely to gain the feeling that the consultation is an ongoing process and that they will have a say in the outcome.

One of the difficult issues for a consultant occurs when they encounter a hostile or passive client. Both of these resistant behaviors are a challenge. Hostile clients may be encountered when the consultee brings such a person in to meet with the consultant. Hostile clients are typically uncooperative and may resent talking with the consultant, feeling that they are being blamed for the problem or just that they have nothing to do with solving the problem. In this situation the consultant tries to understand why the client has such hostility. Does the client recognize that there is such a problem? Does the person feel trapped into being in the consultation? If the consultee is able to understand the client's position, the person may relax and be helpful in the process. If the client is unmanageable, the consultation may have to be discontinued.

Passive clients present problems which may be as difficult to resolve. It is important for everyone involved to present their ideas and to work toward problem solving. Passive clients may be incapable or unwilling to suggest ideas or even freely discuss the problem being presented. This client may not be willing to give an accurate picture of the situation but, unlike the hostile client, may be taking too much responsibility for their role in the problem.

Not all conflict and resistance is negative, however. In fact, when one works through the conflict and resistance, it will pave the way for better solutions. But the consultant must use his or her skills to assure that conflict and resistance do not move into more destructive modes.

Training

The effectiveness of consultation in any setting depends on the expertise of the consultant (Kratochwill and VanSomeren, 1985) and the skill level and motivation of the consultee (Gutkin and Curtis, 1982). The major issue involves whether consultants need specific training in order to consult or if only their work experience in their area of expertise is sufficient. The majority of consultants offer their services without formal training in the consulting process. They are experts in a particular area and offer that advice and service.

Training in consultation has occurred most frequently in short-term training sessions, not full-fledged training programs. Only 33 percent of counselor education programs were found to have a separate course on consulting (Splete and Bernstein, 1981). Training in consultation should include sufficient course work and sufficient supervised field experience

(Meyers, Wurtz, and Flannagan, 1981). This may be difficult for the developing consultant to locate. Both Brown (1985) and Leonard (1977) advocate training to develop specializations or specific consultation competencies. A comprehensive plan that proposes training modalities has been outlined by Brown (1985) and Gibbs (1985). It calls for specific training with a cross-cultural perspective. This would include didactic information about the impact of sociocultural factors in consultation, culturally appropriate intervention strategies, and placement experiences with diverse groups.

There have been many parallels drawn between the training needed for consultation and that needed in a clinical approach (Blanton and Alley, 1978; Brown, Kurpius, and Morris, 1988; Cochran, 1982). Many of the skills used in counseling or in group therapy are transferable to the consulting process. Forming a relationship, collecting data, assessment, diagnosis, and planning interventions are areas in which there are similarities and overlap between the required skills. However, there are also distinct differences in the methods and goals of counseling and consultation (Blanton and Alley, 1978). It behooves the consultant to understand the various approaches to consulting to avoid the tendency to view it and counseling as one and the same.

Gallessich (1962) has said that the concepts and processes of consulting are not well understood. We have only descriptive models and no actual theories; therefore, consultation continues to be performed in varying degrees of effectiveness. She also has pointed out that the consultant's effectiveness is probably not determined by education or intellect but more by interpersonal skills. If the person is skillful in diagnosing and establishing interpersonal relationships, he or she has a possibility of becoming an effective consultant.

There is also the issue of consultee competence and training. Kampwith (1987) identified five impediments to successful consultation with teachers. These same impediments are likely to have an impact with consultees in other work environments as well. Kampwith focused on Caplan's concept of theme interference, indicating that there may be a "lack of objectivity caused by a belief system or bias" (p. 119). He lists the teacher's lack of skills in following through, guilt and defensiveness, and discouragement when the results do not occur quickly as other impediments to consultation. Consultee limitations may well form a barrier to effective consultation despite the skills and efforts of the consultant.

When the consultation involves consultee training, other issues arise. According to Gutkin and Curtis (1982) consultation is effective in making confident persons more confident, but it is of little value to those who may need the help most. This appears to be true in individual as well as in group consulting. In a study of multidisciplinary teams, Flemming and Flemming

(1983) concluded that well-functioning teams were open to the consultation process and benefited from it while at schools where communication between team members was poor, the teams were threatened by the process, they hesitated to admit weaknesses, and changes were minimal. Several researchers have recognized the need for consultee training in the school setting (Kratochwill and VanSomeren, 1985; Gutkin and Curtis, 1982; Gutkin and Bossard, 1984; Anderson, Kratochwill, and Bergan, 1986; Flemming and Flemming, 1983), but there is a difference of opinion on the most effective method. Inservice training focused on behavior management principles and on specific consulting strategies including problem identification, plans, and observational techniques for data collection, and the development of interventions have been demonstrated as effective (Anderson, Kratochwill, and Bergan, 1986).

Cultural Differences

Consultants may find ethnic variations in consultees and clients an issue. Gibbs (1980) found that due to different historical, cultural, and social values and patterns, some difficulty occurred when the consultant was white and the consultee was black. The focus in those consultation relationships was on the interpersonal rather than the content aspects.

Distinct differences exist between how people from different ethnic backgrounds view the consultant and the consultation process. Whatever the race of the consultant, however, minority consultees tend to be more suspicious and reserved (Gibbs, 1980). She states that their focus is on an interpersonal orientation and defines this as "the value of the group or individual which focuses on the process rather than the content of interaction, both verbal and nonverbal, between two people." This is particularly true during the early phase of consultation.

An awareness of ethnic differences may help expedite a resolution of the problem. There is, however, another side to the issue. That is, by expecting differences and acting in subtle ways that may alert the consultee, the consultant may undermine his or her own work. Each situation needs to be judged on its own merit rather than on preconceived sets of notions regarding ethnic differences.

SUMMARY

Mental health consultation generally involves helping solve problems with individuals, groups, or organizations. A consultant needs knowledge about the specific problem area, skill in human relations, and knowledge of various models of consultation. This chapter presented descriptions of the major models. While there are similarities in these models, there are some distinct differences which may make certain models more appropriate for specific problems or more preferred by individual consultants. Later chapters will apply several of these models to consultations in different settings. The chapter ended with an exploration of numerous issues that consultants face. Many of the issues do not have a "right" answer; however, how a consultant behaves in such situations will affect his/her decisions. Reviewing such issues at this point in the book helps in understanding issues in the remaining chapters as well as preparing for the role of consultant.

REFERENCES

ABIDIN, R. R. Negative effects of behavioral consultation. *Journal of School Psychology,* 13, 51–57.

ANDERSON, T., KRATOCHWILL, T., and BERGAN, J. (1986). Training teachers in behavioral consultation therapy: An analysis of verbal behaviors. *Journal of School Psychology,* 24, 229–241.

BABCOCK, N. L., and PRYZWANSKY, W. B. (1983). Models of consultation: Preferences of educational professionals at five stages of service. *Journal of School Psychology,* 21, 359–366.

BANDURA, A. (1969). *Principles of behavioral modification.* New York: Holt, Rinehart and Winston.

BERGAN, J. R. (1977). *Behavioral consultation.* Columbus, OH: Charles E. Merrill Publishing Company.

BLANTON, J., and ALLEY, S. (1978). Clinical and nonclinical aspects of program development consultation. *Professional Psychology,* 5, 315–321.

BROWN, D., KURPIUS, D., and MORRIS, J. (1988). *Handbook of consultation with individuals and small groups.* Association for Counselor Education and Supervision.

CAPLAN, G. (1970). *The theory and practice of mental health consultation.* New York: Basic Books.

CARR, C. (1989). Following through on change. *Training,* 26 (1), 39–44.

DINKMEYER, D., et al. (1984). School counselors as consultants in primary prevention programs. *Personnel and Guidance Journal,* 62, 464–466.

DOUGLAS, J. (1982). A "systems" perspective to behavioral consultation in schools: A personal view. *Bulletin of the British Psychological Society,* 35, 195–197.

FITZGERALD, T. H. (1987). The OD practitioner in the business world: Theory versus reality. *Organizational Dynamics,* 16 (1), 20–33.

FLEMMING, D., and FLEMMING, E. (1983). Consultation with multidisciplinary teams: A program of development in improvement in team functioning. *Journal of School Psychology,* 21, 367–376.

FRANK, L. (1936). Society as the patient. *American Journal of Sociology,* 42, 335–344.

GALLESSICH, J. (1982). *The profession and practice of consultation: A handbook for consultants, trainers of consultants, and consumers of consultation services.* San Francisco: Jossey-Bass.

GALLESSICH, J. (1985). Toward a meta-theory of consultation. *The Counseling Psychologist,* 13, 336–362.

GAUPP, K. (1966). Authority, influence and control in consultation. *Community Mental Health Journal*, 2, 205–210.

GIBBS, J. (1980). The interpersonal orientation in mental health consultation: Toward a model of ethnic variations in consultation. *Journal of Community Psychology*, 8, 195–207.

GLUCKSTERN, N., and PACKARD, R. (1977). The internal–external change agent team: Bringing change to a "closed institution." *Journal of Applied Behavioral Science*, 13, 41–52.

GOODWIN, D. L., and COATES, T. J. (1977). The teacher–pupil interaction scale: An empirical method for analyzing the interactive effects of teacher and pupil behavior. *Journal of School Psychology*, 15, 51–59.

GUTKIN, T., and BOSSARD, M. (1984). The impact of consultant, consultee, and organizational variables on teacher attitudes towards consultation services. *Journal of School Psychology*, 22, 251–258.

GUTKIN, T., and CURTIS, M. (1982). School-based consultations: Theory and techniques. In G. R. Reynolds and T. B. Getkin (eds.), *The handbook of school psychology* (796–828). New York: John Wiley.

HARRISON, R. (1970). Choosing the depth of organization intervention. *Journal of Applied Behavioral Science*, 6 (2), 181–202.

HENGEVELD, M., and ROOYMANS, H. (1983). The relevance of a staff-oriented approach in consultation psychiatry: A preliminary study. *General Psychiatry*, 5, 259–264.

HIRSCHOWITZ, R. G. (1978). Consultation to changing organizations. *Psychiatric Opinion*, 15, 29–33.

JOINT COMMISSION ON MENTAL ILLNESS AND HEALTH. (1961). *Action for Mental Health*. New York: Basic Books.

KAMPWITH, T. (1987). Consultation: Strategy for dealing with children's behavior problems. *Technique: A Journal for Remedial Education and Counseling*, 3, 117–120.

KELNER, F. B. (1984). A rehabilitation approach to program diagnosis in technical assistance consultation. *Psychosocial Rehabilitation Journal*, 7 (3), 32–43.

KRATOCHWILL, T., and VANSOMEREN, K. (1985). Barriers to treatment success in behavioral consultation: Current limitations in future directions. *Journal of School Psychology*, 23, 225–239.

KURPIUS, D. J. (1985). Consultation interventions: Successes, failures and proposals. *The Counseling Psychologist*, 13 (3), 368–389.

LENNOX, N., FLANAGAN, D., and MEYERS, J. (1979). Organizational consultation to facilitate communication within a school staff. *Psychology in the Schools*, 16 (4), 520–526.

LOUNSBURY, J., ROISIUM, K., PAKARNEY, L., SILLS, A., and MEISSEN, G. (1979). An analysis of topic areas and topic trends in the *Community Mental Health Journal* from 1965 through 1977. *Community Mental Health Journal*, 15, 267–276.

LOVELADY, L. (1984). Change strategies and the use of OD consultants to facilitate change. *Leadership and Organizational Development Journal*, 5 (4), 2–12.

MACLENNAN, B., QUINN, R., and SCHROEDER, D. (1975). The scope of community mental health consultation. In F. Mannino, B. MacLennan, and M. Shore (eds.), *The practice of mental health consultation* (DHEW Publication No. ADM 74-112) (3–24). Washington, DC: U.S. Government Printing Office.

MARTIN, R., and MEYERS, J. (1980). School psychologists and the practice of consultation. *Psychology in the Schools*, 17, 478–484.

MEYERS, J., WURTZ, R., and FLANNAGAN, D. (1981). A national survey investigating consultation training occurring in school psychology programs. *Psychology in the Schools,* 18, 297–302.

NUFRIO, P. M. (1983). Diary of a mad internal consultant. *Group and Organization Studies,* 8, 7–14.

PARSONS, R. D., and MEYERS, J. (1984). *Developing consultation skills.* San Francisco: Jossey-Bass.

POLLEY, R. B. (1987). The consultant as the shaper of legend. *Consultation,* 6 (2), 102–118.

RUSSELL, M. L. (1978). Behavioral consultation: Theory and process. *Personnel and Guidance Journal,* 2, 346–350.

SATTLER, J. (1982). *Assessment of children's intelligence and special abilities,* 2nd ed. Boston: Allyn and Bacon.

SCHEIN, E. (1978). The role of the consultant: Content expert or process facilitator? *Personnel and Guidance Journal,* 56, 339–343.

SCHEIN, E. (1969). *Process consultation: Its role in organization development.* Reading, MA: Addison-Wesley.

SPLETE, H., and BERNSTEIN, B. (1981). A survey of consultation training as a part of counselor education programs. *Personnel and Guidance Journal,* 3, 470–472.

STEELE, F. (1969). Consultants and detectives. *The Journal of Applied Behavioral Science,* 5, 187–202.

WHITE, P. L., and FINE, M. J. (1976). The effects of three school psychological consultation modes on selected teacher and pupil outcomes. *Psychology in the Schools,* 13 (4), 414–420.

YEAGER, J. (1982). Managing executive performance: The corporate private practice. *Professional Psychology,* 13, 587–593.

CHAPTER TWO
PROCESS
AND PROCEDURES
OF CONSULTING

There are numerous models and procedures in consultation. This may be because each consultant is a product of a unique set of experiences leading to differences in their concepts and approaches. Cherniss (1978) suggested that problems in consultation result from a lack of solid theoretical base and from the variation in consultation terminology and reporting methods. Many individual consultants lack clear conceptual directions, and individual consulting styles have not been well integrated into a general framework (Dworkin and Dworkin, 1975). Therefore, individuals wishing to apply consulting methods are likely to be confronted with a mass of information that does not provide a basic set of procedures. On closer examination, however, most of the procedures in consultation follow a similar set of stages of planning, entry, diagnosis, goal setting, implementation, evaluation, maintenance, withdrawal, and follow-up (Redmon, Cullari, and Farris, 1985).

Consultation procedures can be described in terms of behaviors which cut across individual models. The consultation process is a set of stages and procedures that are general enough to encompass most models and identify the behaviors that are part of each stage. Describing the numerous but similar methods, we can make data from a variety of sources more compatible. This chapter will present the process and procedures of consultations in five stages: preentry, initial contact and relationship establishment, assessment and diagnosis, intervention, and termination. Although some procedures may vary, these stages are generally followed in consulting with both individuals and organizations. Later chapters will illustrate some variations in procedures; however, the following stages appropriately prepare the reader for the remaining chapters.

PREENTRY

The consultation process begins prior to entering a consulting relationship. In this stage the consultant examines and defines values, assumptions, and needs about people, work, and organizations. Questions regarding one's views on personal authority, power, position, and competencies need to be answered. What are the beliefs held about organizational structure, purpose, and the use of reward and punishment (Kurpius, 1978)? Preentry is a time of training and preparation for the developing consultant.

The consultant, if effective, will be in a position of influence and the belief system adopted will determine the manner in which the consultation occurs. The conceptualization of the problem that the consultant is called on to help remedy is dependent on one's beliefs and assumptions.

Gallessich (1985) looks at five dimensions of variability in the deliverance of consulting services. Conceptualization of the problem depends on the depth and breadth with which problems are defined. Whether the problem is viewed independently or in the context of the social structure, whether the problem is seen as a result of knowledge deficits or of the presence of personality variables, the conceptualization will provide potency in regard to decisions on the other dimensions: goals, methods and assumptions (locus and strategies), consultant role, and values. Becoming clear on one's personal assumptions about the roots of a problem and how change occurs is essential prior to becoming a consultant.

For example, one who looks at a presenting problem in a systems context will have a different assessment, method of intervention, and goal than the consultant who conceptualizes in terms of personality variables or capacities. If one assumes that the role of the consultant is educative and not prescriptive, the intervention will vary in ways affecting length and nature of contact. Whether one sees him/herself as a content expert or as a process expert will provide an orientation for the intervention.

If the consultant assumes that the consultee is in need of a prescription for alleviating a problem, a solution is generally provided. This intervention is at great variance from the consultant who assumes that one's role is an educative one in which consultees can determine their own solution given certain knowledge. These differing conceptualizations, assumptions, and values often determine the consultation model adopted by the consultant, that is, educative or organizational.

Cherniss (1976) operationalizes the stage of preentry in terms of three questions. The first question is, "Should I do consultation in this situation?" When a consultee poses the problem and requests services from the consultant, the consultant needs to ask for enough information to decide whether she/he wishes to enter this relationship. The second and third questions clearly relate to that decision. The second question is, "Whose interests are being met?" The consultant needs to determine the competing interests of the individuals and groups and to assess how these will impact on the potential for successful consultation. The third question, "What is the focus of the consultation?" involves the consultant's estimates of the level and the extent of the intervention that is necessary for success. A discussion of these three questions with the consultee is imperative at this pre-entry stage. The consultant may also want to have a second meeting with other individuals involved in the consultation situation. This may involve other administrators or members of the board of education, if working with a school, or the board of directors of an agency or company. Such a meeting enhances knowledge for the consultant and makes the consultees aware of the consultant's perspective of what may be needed and what will occur in the consultation process.

The consultant needs to have access to all information pertaining to the problem. When possible, the consultant should read documents about the organization, study the problem area, and discuss the political behavior of the consultee's staff. This information is helpful in determining if the environment is likely to be supportive as well as in preparing for specific problems in the initial, formal contact.

O'Neill and Trickett (1982) emphasize the compatibility between the consultant and consultee. Compatibility often includes some similarity in training and experience as well as of values and beliefs. Although some differences are to be expected, strong differences in the manner in which the consultant and consultee look at problems and the general philosophy of problem solutions could cause difficulty.

By the end of the preentry stage, the consultant should have studied the characteristics of the consultee, assessed compatibility, determined the available resources necessary to support the intervention, and made a decision whether the consultation is likely to be successful and whether to continue (Redmon et al., 1985).

In summary, preentry is a time for the consultant to examine his orientation and beliefs, which will shape the manner in which service is provided. It is necessary to clarify one's position so that it can be articulated to the consultee, in order to determine if there is agreement in the conceptualization of the problem and the designing of interventions. Developing consultants need to familiarize themselves with various approaches and models of consultation in order to be effective helpers. Specific training and practice in the field under supervision facilitate the development of consultation competency.

INITIAL CONTACT

During this stage the consultant first has contact with the consultee. The tasks at hand include: (1) assess the readiness for change and intervention; (2) develop a working relationship; and (3) develop an understanding of the consultee's situation/problem and work climate. It is also a time to determine the expectations and purpose of the consultation, any hidden agendas, the compatibility of the consultant's skills with the consultee's problems; to define and agree upon the roles of the parties; and to formulate both written and psychological contracts. The consultant's first contact is generally initiated by the consultee for one of several reasons: to prevent an anticipated problem, to remediate an existing difficulty, or to facilitate and promote individual or group growth.

Kahn and Mann (1959) presented initial contact in terms of three categories: single, dual, and multiple. The labels refer to the number of levels or groups within a consultee organization. Clearly, if the consultant is only going to meet with one teacher, set of parents, or one manager of an organization for an individual consultation, there is, in reality, only one level. Even so, teachers may not be able to resolve the problem or carry out the consultation alone if it involves more than control within their classroom. Parents are sometimes unable to carry out interventions without cooperation between each other or the family system, and frequently one employee cannot successfully carry out interventions without assistance from other levels or persons within the organization. Kahn and Mann suggest that when two or more factions are involved, the consultant makes the initial contact with all levels at once so that no one is left out. Such a simultaneous contact can be important because the first contact often influences both the consultant and consultee. It may, however, not be possible. Frequently the consultant is contacted by only one person in a system. If the consultant is going to deal with a dual or multiple entry, he or she needs to have identified the functional levels within this consultee hierarchy in advance. In working with an organization, the consultant may be able to meet with the formal group, such as the administration, the line staff, and possibly representatives of other formal organizations. Even so, informal groups may present resistance if they are not represented by the formal hierarchy.

Redmon and colleagues (1985) proposed several steps for the consultant during the initial period: (1) Identify all levels to be involved in the consulation prior to planning any intervention. (2) Make sure that all levels are represented or notified when the initial contact is made. (3) If the consultant meets with one level privately, the same opportunity should be extended to other levels in the consultee system. (4) The consultant should communicate the conditions of the consultation to all levels of consultees. This information should include who asked for the consultation and for what reasons. (5) All representatives should have a role in the planning of interventions from the beginning. (6) The consultant needs to establish a psychological contact that permits flexibility in examining the context of the consultation and yet helps to clarify the goals and personal desires between the consultee and consultant. It is important to negotiate a formal contract that specifies the timeline and costs and provides descriptions of any legal details.

During this initial stage some level of agreement on the course of the consultation is required. O'Neill and Trickett (1982) suggest the consultant negotiate a contract that permits some exploration before expectations are established. Schein (1969) has suggested that two types of contracts need to be considered. The formal contract determines the amount of time spent by the consultant, the services provided, and the fee, and stipulates that either party can terminate with appropriate notice. The psychological contract concerns the general relationship between the consultant and consultee. This defines what the consultee wishes to gain from the arrangement as well as the nature and extent of the consultant's expectations of the consultee. If these are not thoroughly explored prior to establishing the formal contract, either or both participants may be disappointed. One psychological component important in the contract has to do with confidentiality and whether staff evaluation is a part of consultation. Although the consultee may not mention this, an administrator may expect the consultant to provide feedback regarding the effectiveness of staff, and these data could be used to retain or not retain certain staff members. That worry keeps many staff members from being open and, therefore, interferes with the assessment the consultant needs to determine an appropriate intervention.

Assessing Readiness for Change

The initiation of a consulting relationship presumes that the consultant has genuine interest in working in the consultee environment. The consulting relationship requires interaction; empathy for the consultee and his work environment is a necessary precondition to the process. An issue related to the determination of a good "match" is whether the consultant has sufficient knowledge of the client's milieu and the skills necessary to act as a change agent in that work environment. In the following example, the consultant comes to some important conclusions that help illustrate this dimension.

> A consultant is contacted to help remedy a staff problem in a juvenile court system by the court director. In the initial meeting they let it be known that they see themselves in terms of a dysfunctional family who needs therapy. The consultant, on the other hand, holds to a model which will facilitate the staff learning how to problem solve, which will ultimately reduce the need for further consultations. In further dialogue with the staff it becomes clear that they are not open to other methods of intervention and the consultant indicates an inability to provide service.

In this scenario, the consultant might conclude that the staff, as a whole, is not willing to explore the possibilities for change. If the consultant views himself as a process facilitator and a change agent who relies on collaboration, assuming the role of a counselor who uses family systems techniques is not congruent. In either assessment, the conclusion would be the same: consultation would likely be ineffective.

The consultee will have identified a need for assistance at the time of contact, which indicates a readiness for intervention and a desire for change. Leaving the initiation of contact to the consultee, the consultant usually can presuppose readiness to work toward finding a solution to a problem. However, it is important to assess the readiness for change on whatever level intervention is sought. The success of the process will depend to a large extent on the degree of openness the consultee exhibits as well as the congruence between the consultant and consultees.

In another example, a therapist involved in the treatment of a particularly difficult client seeks consultation. It can be presumed she wants intervention and suggestions by the consultant. In another case, a plant manager might contract for consultation regarding his employee training program. However, will the personnel who would be responsible for implementing any changes be as willing to consider recommendations? In the initial contact, the consultant's relationship and assessment skills will be used in seeking answers to several questions. Is there a willingness to explore why situations or problems exist? More importantly, is there a willingness to change if change is necessary?

Often consultation is not effective because what the consultee desires is removal of a problem rather than help in dealing with one. There may not be a commitment for change until a crisis situation develops (Berger, 1979). A receptive attitude on the part of the consultee who will be implementing any recommendations is crucial to the successful consultation and needs to be thoroughly examined by the consultant. Beyond making a mental note, the consultant needs to discuss the implications for change, determine readiness, and be able to outline the roles of the parties in the process.

Establishing the Relationship

One of the first steps in consulting requires that the consultant outline to the consultee the tasks involved. This needs to be done in an atmosphere that contributes to the establishment of a helping relationship, one in which there is freedom from interuptions. As in any other helping relationship, eye contact and body posture facilitate the communication between the consultee and consultant. Relationship skills transfer and are applicable to the establishment of a good working alliance between the consultant and the consultee.

There are several consultant attitudes and agendas which appear to facilitate a good working relationship. The relationship is of crucial importance. There is little confidence in any advice or suggestions when there is no opportunity to establish a relationship (Koocher, Sourkes, and Keane, 1979). Exploring each other's expectations and needs within the consulting relationship promotes personal trust (Walz and Benjamin, 1978; Westbrook, Leonard, Johnson, Boyd, Hunt, and McDermott, 1978; Russ, 1978).

The consulting relationship, as with other helping relationships, is comprised of the core helping conditions of empathy, respect, genuineness, and concreteness (Carkhuff, 1983). The consultant can reduce any tendency towards defensiveness on the part of the consultee by acknowledging that the consultee's contribution to the process is essential for success. By demonstrating he/she values and understands the consultee's tasks and recognizes the consultee's need to familiarize the consultant with the job situation, the consultant gives the consultee permission to express and clarify needs (Lamb and Peterson, 1983). He/she also demonstrates empathy for the position of the consultee.

Parsons and Meyers (1984) make several specific recommendations that increase the likelihood of developing a collegial consulting relationship: (1) Allow the consultee the option of accepting or rejecting consultee suggestions. (2) Promote consultee's contributions to solution sets. (3) Encourage consultee decision-making behaviors. (4) Acknowledge and highlight consultee contributions. (5) Promote the acceptance of responsibility by the consultee. (6) Require effort from the consultee.

The consultation alliance is seen by Russ (1978) as one of the two key variables in effective consulting, the other being facilitation of information processing. The parallels between the consultation alliance and other types of helping relationships are evident. First, a consultant holds the expectation that change is possible and views the consultee as significant in the process, and the consultee is able to see his/her own potential for being effective. Second, in a safe relationship between the two parties, there is likely to be greater risk taking on the part of the consultee in terms of problem-solving thoughts and actions. Third, a strong consultation alliance facilitates the exploration of attitudes and subtle influences on the problem situation. Finally, the mirroring of problem-solving behavior by the consultee is more likely to occur if the consultant has become significant to the consultee and respect exists.

Contracting

We need to attend to the structuring of the relationship on two levels and in several dimensions. There are two levels on which structuring occurs: explicit and implicit. An example of explicit structure is when either party refers to their role in the relationship, a reference that generally implies the power position of that role (Brown, Kurpius, and Morris, 1988). It can occur at the onset of the relationship when the consultant outlines how he views consultation (i.e., as a collaborative endeavor). Such structuring can also come from the consultee in expressing agreements or compromises on what role each is to play. Implicit structure then follows, since the consultant would insure that interventions or other aspects of the process reflect this agreed-upon collaborative effort (Brown, Kurpius, and Morris, 1988). This process of structuring or affirming the roles of the parties continues in the dialogue throughout the consultation process.

Structuring the power of the relationship is just one aspect of the contracting process. Other dimensions may be structured more formally. They include setting the times (including perhaps a timeline) for consultation, the location where service will be provided, fees and costs, how services will be evaluated and by whom, and the roles and responsibilities of both the consultant and consultee in the problem-solving process. Such contracting makes explicit the consulting process structure.

Although it is not always necessary to have a written contract, it can be advantageous. The contract should be based on mutual collaboration and should specify the purpose of the consultation, role of the consultant and consultee, and work setting. With these basics understood, the process tends to flow smoothly and exploring the problem becomes easier.

Understanding the Problem Situation

This step in the initial stage has overlap with the previous steps, determining the readiness for change and developing the consulting relationship. In the process of assessment and developing a collegial relationship, the consultee's conceptualization of the problem will become evident. The reason for the consultee's seeking consultation should be given as sharp a focus as possible.

This is an area ripe for potential problems. There may be hidden agendas or purposes not articulated by the consultee. The better the relationship and trust, the more likely that the consultee will be honest in presenting the problem and the true purpose of desiring intervention.

Another pitfall is that as the relationship develops, personal disclosures may increase. It is imperative that the consultant refocus the energy on the problem or the consultation could develop into therapy. A technique called supportive refocusing (Randolph, 1985) may be used when the focus has shifted to a personal dilemma of the consultee. The consultant recognizes the consultee's problem and expresses empathy while at the same time shifting attention to assisting the consultee with the problem at hand. If therapy is indicated, the consultant has the option of giving the consultee a referral.

In providing a sharp focus on the reason for consultation, the consultee's conception of the difficulties and definition of the issues will be given top priority. This not only communicates that the consultant is interested in helping but, when the consultant shows appreciation for the consultee's contribution, it strengthens the relationship. It may be important for the consultant to become familiar with the work milieu of the factory, the policies of the police force, or the specific classroom situation of a teacher, depending on the consultee's work environment.

Identifying whether the focus is on short- or long-term remediation, problem prevention, or growth enhancement may help determine the type of assessment and diagnosis needed to plan interventions. It may dictate whether the consultant uses the "expert" or content model, the process model (Schien, 1969), the collaborative mode (Kurpuis, 1978), or any one of several models of consultation mentioned earlier. To some extent, the model employed may be a result of the bias of the consultant. The consultant must be aware of various theoretical models of consultation to ensure that issues are getting the most appropriate attention and mediation.

It is important that the consultant demonstrate that the relationship desired is a collegial one. Rather than beginning with a diagnostic stance, the consultant's role is that of an appreciative visitor who is willing to acknowledge the strengths and tasks of the consultee and the organization. Any subtle communication that the consultant views the consultee as incompetent will obviously impair the building of a collaborative relationship. The consultant must also be aware of any overt or unconscious tendency for the consultee to feel that the consultant should assume full responsibility for the problem remediation. The consultant does not have the resources or power to solve the problem alone.

The assistance of the consultee in the next stage of the consultation process is crucial. Unless the foundations for the helping relationship have been laid during the initial contact stage, subsequent contacts will be lacking and the chances for a "successful" consultation will decrease. Again, it is in this initial stage that determination of attitudes toward change are begun, that the roles and expectations are formed, the relationship established, and movement toward problem resolution begins.

ASSESSMENT AND DIAGNOSIS

The process of assessment and diagnosis begins during the preentry stage and is ongoing until termination. It occurs during the entire consultation process. For example, in the stages already discussed there were several points where assessment was necessary. However, there are specific tasks in this stage which must be addressed before moving along in the consultation process. Goodstein (1978) summarized Argyris's (1970) treatment of diagnosis by identifying three important steps in that process: developing information, helping the consultee to examine alternatives, and facilitating internal commitment. Data is collected either by the consultant or by others for the consultant to determine exactly what the problem is or to verify the problem as reported by the consultee. When the problem is clearly defined and agreed upon by the consultee and consultant, they can quickly examine strategies of resolution. Cooperative discussions are important groundwork in reaching a diagnosis that agrees exactly on the nature of the problem. Continued cooperation then is used to establish goals and to select a procedure to follow. The final step in diagnosis involves developing a commitment of the consultee that will influence the remaining stages of consultation. It is important that the consultee see the final direction as an effective solution and provide sufficient resources to that approach.

Gathering Data

The purpose of collecting data is to pinpoint and clarify the problem areas that the consultee has identified. There may be times when the problem definition might change as a consequence of gathering and analyzing the data. The consultant who knows several models of consultation will be able to tailor these methods within the milieu of the consultee. A knowledgeable consultant will also be familiar with several systems of classifying data and of diagnosis, for example, behavioral, developmental, or systemic.

Brown, Kurpius, and Morris (1988) note two criteria to be used when selecting a system. First, the consultant needs to be able to thoroughly explain the system used to the consultee. Second, there needs to be acceptance of the system on the part of the consultee. If there is resistance to one system, another can be suggested by the perceptive consultant.

In respect to role definition within this step, the contract should specify who will collect, synthesize, and analyze the data in order to diagnose the problem. Another issue is related to the methods of data collection, of which there are several. The innumerable ways to conceptually interpret the data gathered will in some part influence the intervention agreed upon.

It is important to remember that misinterpretation of the data, or a bias toward a certain outcome, will negatively influence the decisions that will be made in regard to the target for intervention. Thus, both parties must be open to examining several variables which might impact the problem area and refrain from imposing their preliminary conceptualization on the process. As a guard against data misuse and to provide maximum information to both the consultant and consultee, gathering and reviewing the data as a shared task is recommended.

One source of consultee resistance which might be encountered during this step has been observed by Piersel and Gutkin (1983). They note that the consultee's anxiety increases when faced with the possibility that the consultant will uncover additional problems. Randolph and Graun (1988) believe that this anxiety might be heightened when the consultant chooses to observe the consultee in the work setting. When the consultant makes himself equally vulnerable (i.e., models risk-taking behavior by demonstrating alternative strategies and inviting consultee critique), Randolph (1985) believes that the consultee's anxiety is moderated. Data gathering may be threatening to the consultee, and it is the wise consultant who recognizes and discusses this issue.

Some of the more common methods to collect data include observation, surveys, checklists, interviews, background information, and review of standardized records. The factors which influence the methods of collection include the model, the nature of the consultee (individual, group, or organization), and the problem initially identified. Questions to be answered include: What is the history of this problem? When did it start? How long has it been occurring? What is the impact? What interventions or solutions have already been tried? Which produced results? Why weren't previous attempts (if there were any) successful? What information is needed to come to a better understanding of these issues? These questions guide the manner in which data are collected.

Diagnosis

Like some of the previous steps, diagnosis and data collection are ongoing. Careful diagnosis leaves room for the incorporation of new information in the conceptualization of the problem. The actual process of diagnosis has to be carefully determined. The original conceptualization of the problem lies in the mind of the consultee.

In coming to a definition of the problem, both the consultant and the consultee need to have a shared understanding of the issues. In this respect, there are parallels to the client–therapist relationship: the client may come in with an initial problem, but in gathering background data both may come to a new understanding of what needs to be addressed. Likewise, the therapist may sometimes want to make interpretations and other times ask questions of the client so that the client may arrive at his own discoveries. Regardless of the client issue, the competent therapist will have a systematic method of assessment and diagnosis, dependent on the theoretical orientation used to view the client.

The system used by the consultant is similar. It guides the diagnostic process by outlining the salient questions to be addressed. A system of diagnosis provides a way to classify consultee problems. The target of diagnosis is different from a therapist: the target in consultation is on problem or task resolution. Unless the consultee participates in the diagnostic process by arriving at some notions of how problems developed (this discovery coming from new data or by subtle interventions by the consultant) and what needs resolution, the investment in the process of change is reduced. A lack of investment contributes to resistance or low motivation in the implementation of solution strategies. Generally, the consultant is viewed as either a content or process expert. Within these two roles, there are several diagnostic systems that one might employ, for example behavioral, systemic, or humanistic.

Suppose a consultant is hired to provide assistance to an elementary classroom teacher who is having difficulty with a student. The teacher notes that the student is having problems remaining in his seat and is being disruptive to his classmates. It is reported that neither attempts to punish nor ignoring the behavior has produced results.

In considering the example of a behavioral system for analyzing data and diagnosis, there are several categories of information needed. Berger (1977) suggests obtaining baseline data to determine the frequency of the problem behavior and locating environmental factors which contribute or reinforce the behavior. This would include observing what behavior precedes the student leaving his seat, determining under what circumstances that behavior does or does not occur, and whether it happens with his other teachers. In this case, the goal would be to devise interventions to reduce the incidence of out-of-seat behavior from the baseline measure taken prior to intervention.

A systems approach for diagnosis of this same problem would necessitate gathering data related to the student's interactions with the teacher and other students, school personnels' attitudes towards the student, and the relationship between home and school (Douglas, 1982). Other data would include recognition of any specific problem of the student, for example a learning disability, and how it affects not only teacher expectations of the child but the motivational level of the teacher and support from other staff to try alternatives. The out-of-seat behavior would be seen in the context of the student's background and the totality of the home and school experience. Like the behavioral system, some measure of the behavior might be taken to determine the effectiveness of treatment strategies.

Gallessich (1982) describes another conceptual strategy called "open systems approach." A way to evaluate and diagnose agency problems, it includes factoring in history, societal mandates and community expectations, goals and underlying values, inputs from clients and staff, and consideration for funding and materials. In addition, the structure of the agency is examined as well as the service delivery, communication patterns, decision-making process, and attitudes of staff. Interactions between the agency and other professional organizations as well as political considerations are reviewed. Within this framework, determining the focus for intervention will still necessitate the adoption of a theoretical base to explain why certain conditions exist and what can be done to impact the problem areas.

When the consultant is working in a large system, there may be differing definitions of the problem areas. An administrator might have one conceptualization and the staff another. The goals of the parties may differ, and it will become problematic when evaluating the success of the consultation if there is no movement towards shared assumptions by all parties. Without agreement on what the problems are, there can be no consensus on the goals or interventions for change. Lennox, Flannagan, and Meyers (1979) suggest utilizing feedback sessions and surveys to reduce any resistance that might be encountered here and reach a shared understanding of positions.

Other focus areas for consultee problems are outlined by Blake and Mouton (1978) and Caplan (1970). Four major focal issues are provided by Blake and Mouton, who note that the consultee's issue may be any of the four, or a combination of them. These focal points are: (1) the exercise of power and authority, (2) moral and cohesion difficulties, (3) problems arising from holding standards or norms of conduct, and (4) problematic goals or objectives. Caplan sees problems arising from one of four possible areas: lack of understanding, not possessing the necessary knowledge or skill to resolve issues, lack of objectivity about one's situation, or not feeling competent to resolve an issue. This conceptualization can also guide the data collection and diagnostic process as it suggests areas for review and deficits to be corrected with interventions.

Whatever theoretical construct might be used in counseling can also be used in developing a diagnostic system in consultation as a method to explain or interpret behaviors. It provides a guideline as to what to look for, what type of information is needed, and what type of target areas for intervention strategies might be appropriate.

Goal Setting

The process of goal setting and planning often is a continuation of the diagnostic step. The task involves the final clarification and definition of the problem or interaction of several variables. It is at this point that the problem statement is translated into a goal statement. This transition is actually the most important part of reaching a solution. The consultant and consultee explore the many facets of the problem and all possible variables.

The role of the consultant in setting goals varies from very active to nondirective. In using a behavioral consultation model, the consultant makes the plan and takes primary responsibility in establishing goal statements and procedures. With less directive methods the consultant may serve as a resource, discussing alternatives, or even as a facilitator and have the consultee explore and establish the goals based on their joint diagnosis. Whatever the level of involvement, Redmon and colleagues (1985) list several facets of goal setting and procedure selection that are important: (1) The consultant must describe or help the consultee describe the problem. (2) The consultant must suggest or help the consultee in developing a set of goals and procedures for each goal. (3) The consultant must state the rationale for each goal in terms of the original problem. Each goal must be related to the specific problem. (4) The consultant must include as many involved people as possible in this process. (5) The consultant should summarize these goals and procedures in written form in order to maintain the focus of consultation.

A common method of analysis and diagnosis involves prioritizing the information collected jointly with the consultee and then using a gap theory (Lovelady, 1984). The gap theory involves a point A—identified by the question "Where are we now?"—which is determined by the data gathered and the diagnosis. The consultee and consultant then discuss a state B, which is "Where do we want to be?" The gap is the space between A and B. The challenge is, "How to move from A to B?"

Two other features of goal setting must be considered in the process: determining the impact of the proposed change (or goal attainment) on the environment and outlining the situational variables that accompany the problem resolution (Parsons and Meyers, 1984). By making these assessments, one can evaluate the impact on the system and allow for resultant issues to be addressed initially rather than having one solution set produce a problem down the line. This requires the consultant to be familiar with the program or system of the consultee, and to be cognizant of the practical realities, both positive and negative. These might be issues of resources, time, or even personal variables of the consultee.

Once the specific goals have been established and general procedures outlined, a task analysis should be done, skills evaluated, and roles assigned to individuals who are going to carry out the intervention. Each task necessary to carry out the proposed plan must be described and a time estimated for each step. The result is a list of tasks with a probable time of completion. Each person involved in carrying out an intervention should be assigned a portion of the work. In working with an organization, the consultant tries to avoid the direct intervention. Even when the consultant does assume some role in the intervention process, plans to transfer that responsibility to a regular staff member must be established so the staff can carry on the process after the consultant has terminated from the project.

This can also be a time for resistance on the part of the consultee as the process is moving towards problem resolution. Two possible sources include: (1) incongruent expectations and goals of the consultant and consultee and (2) secondary gain on the part of the consultee from having a problem (Randolph and Graun, 1988). It may be a time to review the initial contract to determine the reason for discrepancies in expectations. Using the relationship to explore and overcome the resistance to previously agreed-upon concepts is important. In exploring the secondary gain of the consultee, arranging contingencies to reduce this can be done on a behavioral-principles level (Randolph and Graun, 1988).

One of the more important aspects of goal setting is to devise a timeline. It provides a way to measure the progress of the interventions agreed upon later. Another essential ingredient is that goals be stated in measurable terms in order to determine the success of the intervention. If, for example, the problem has been defined as one of staff morale, improvement in morale would have to be stated in terms of measurable behaviors, for instance, reduction in absenteeism, improved employee retention rates, or less incidence of union and administrative conflicts. The morale problem would be stated in terms of behaviors that are problematic and lead to the original diagnosis.

Without goal consensus, consultation is doomed. Attention to previous steps in the consultation process can increase the likelihood of shared goals. When the consultant and consultee have established a collaborative relationship, communication is open and there is understanding between the parties as to how the problem is conceptualized. If there has been agreement in how the problems are diagnosed, that is, if there is a shared notion of how difficulties have developed and what is necessary to remedy them, a meeting of the minds should result in terms of goals.

Redmon and colleagues (1985) summarized the processes of carrying out an assessment and diagnosis as (1) data being collected and verified to report on the nature of the problem, (2) assisting the consultee in describing the problem, (3) considering alternative solutions and their consequences, and (4) establishing an approach toward resolution. The consultant must assess and facilitate the consultee's commitment toward the mutually agreed-upon course of action.

INTERVENTION

In selecting interventions it is important to keep the hoped-for results in the forefront of consideration. As in other stages, there must be mutual agreement on the interventions to be employed. The tasks in this stage are to identify options, determining a course of action and implementation of the plan. The groundwork for consensual decision making has been laid in the previous stages of consultation. It is in the intervention stage that the initial problem, if accurately diagnosed, should be reduced or eliminated. The consultant's role is that of resource person, with the consultee needing to shoulder the responsibility for implementing the plan for problem resolution.

It is important that the consultant understand both the breadth and the specificity of an intervention. Argyrs (1970) defined intervention as a method of entering into an ongoing system of relationships, to come between or among individuals, groups, or objects in an effort to help them. Carkhuff (1983) offered an operational definition: that an intervention is both a response and an initiative. It is a response to a deficit or to a situation that has a need while at the same time it is an initiative to influence that situation and transform the deficits into action.

Interventions can be preventative, problem solving, or developmental in scope. Interventions can occur at an individual level, a group level, or an organizational level. As much depends on the training, skills, and orientation of the consultant as it does the context of the consultation, whether it be a classroom, a hospital, or a prison setting. It may be useful to keep these levels and goals of interventions in mind when developing possible strategies.

Identifying Options

Determining the possible angles for responding to the problem area requires some creativity and knowledge about the limitations and resources in the milieu in which the consultation occurs (Lamb and Peterson, 1983). With the assistance of the consultee, a full range of treatment options, interventions, programs, and practices which might positively impact the target areas can be identified as options and opportunities. Balancing the need to identify options with the need to proceed to the action phase is important. Options must be feasible or frustration results. When the consultee has no voice in determining intervention strategies, an opportunity to acquire skills for subsequent use outside of the problem area is lost. Involving the consultee in identifying strategies also lessens the possibility of feeling threatened by the consulting process.

It is important to identify several options so that some choice is possible, lessening the feeling that the consultee was "forced" to act in a defined manner. The consultee needs a voice in the choice, but once that choice has been made, a firm commitment to see it through is necessary. The previous identified sources of resistance may need review by the consultant if consultees are having difficulty generating options.

Classification of Interventions

There are numerous classifications of interventions. The purpose of the classification systems is to provide the consultant and consultee with a broad perspective of possible interventions. The selections of the intervention are not based on the consultant imposing a favorite technique but on selecting the approach that addresses the specific need of the situation. Kurpius (1985) suggested that each intervention is appropriate to "(1) a particular context; (2) a diagnosed human, community or organizational need; (3) a specific target group; and (4) a consultant's values and knowledge of intervention." The consultant chooses the most appropriate intervention by comparing the advantages and disadvantages of the possibilities.

Harrison (1970) provided a classification of interventions based on the depth or the degree of the emotional involvement of the individual in the change process. The four levels of depth are operational analysis, evaluating and controlling individual performance, concern with work style, and interpersonal relationships. In choosing the most appropriate intervention, Harrison suggested the consultant intervene only at the level necessary to produce solutions to the problems and to intervene no deeper than a level at which the energy and resources of the organization can be committed.

Schmuck and Miles (1971) presented a three-dimension classification of interventions. The first, diagnosed problems, includes problems related to the goals, communication, leadership, problem solving, decision making, conflict resolution, and role definition. The second dimension, focusing attention, concentrates on the person, role, diad/triad, intergroup, and total organization. The third dimension, the mode of intervention, is related to the type of intervention (e.g., training, process consultation, confrontation, feedback, problem solving, planning, and technostructural activity).

French and Bell (1973) offer a classification system based on the size and complexity of the consultee organization. For example, with an individual the intervention would include role analysis, life and career planning, and sensitivity training. Consultation with diads or triads would focus on improving the interpersonal relationships through process consultation and third-party consultation. In working with teams and groups, the consultation would focus on team building, survey feedback, group goal setting, and t-groups. When working with intergroup relations, the consultant would use process or task directed intergroup activities. In consulting with a total organization, the consultant would need to examine the structure of the organization and use socio/techno approaches, planning meetings, and survey feedback.

Beer's (1980) classification of major interventions involves a category of diagnostic methods and three categories for interventions which affect one element of the organizational model. The first category focuses on diagnostic interventions such as gathering data about the system and its parts and creating a readiness for feedback and diagnosis. The second category involves process interventions that include activities that help individuals and groups examine their behavior and relationships and move toward better group development. The third category focuses on structural interventions and includes tasks to improve organizational effectiveness by changing the structure. The fourth category includes interventions such as selecting, training, and developing individuals to improve the personal and social-system matching. Beer's classification system is directed toward changing the organization by focusing on training and educating individuals and direct intervention in the social process of the organization or changing the structure of the organization.

Kurpius (1985) and Brown, Kurpius, and Morris (1988) have described three categories of interventions as directed toward the individual, group, and organization. The individual interventions identified by Kurpius include cognitive–behavioral problem solving, life and career interventions, interpersonal–third-party consultation, transactional analysis, and training and development. Group interventions include process consultation, group development and team building, intergroup development, quality circles, and sensitivity-training laboratories. Organizational interventions include human resource development (HRD), survey feedback/action research, organization culture building, strategic planning and choices, job design/enrichment, and management by objective.

Fuqua and Newman (1985) differentiate individual consultation from consulting with a system and focus specifically on the process with an individual. They identify the setting and situations in which individual consultation is most appropriate. These are: when the underlying problem is of an individual nature, when systems interventions would be untimely or unlikely, when perceptions of the problems are limited to individuals, when the system is highly resistant to change, and when individual behavior change is considered more efficient in terms of the present condition of the system. Fuqua and Newman also acknowledge some of the difficult issues encountered in individual consultation. They state that an individual intervention may serve to limit the problem ownership and that individual consultees are likely to generate fewer interventions than a larger system could. Individual consultation emphasizes the consultant's role and responsibility in both problem analysis and resolution activities.

Four possible contexts in which individual consultation might be applied include individual consultation, progression, adaptation, and organizational consultation. Individual consultation can occur when both individual and organization believe the problem is the individual's, and the focus will be on the individual requesting the consultation. An individual may see the problem as an individual responsibility while the organization perceives it as a system problem. Fuqua and Newman describe this as a progression in which consultation moves from an individual perspective to a systems perspective in problem definition and intervention. When an organization perceives a problem as the individual's but the individual believes it is an organization problem, an adaptation type of consultation intervention is required. Obviously, it is more complicated for a system or organization to adapt to the individual characteristics than it is for the individual consultee to adapt to the system's perspective. This may present an interesting consultation situation for the consultant. When both the individual and organization believe the problem is the system situation, organizational intervention is most appropriate. In such a situation the individual is more likely to be a representative of the system at the entry phase of the consultation rather than the specific focus of the consultation.

Blake and Mouton (1978) outline five basic interventions: acceptance, catalyst, confrontation, perscription, and theory and principle. The consultant's acceptance is used to give the consultee a sense of personal security necessary in establishing the working relationship. The consultee feels free to express personal thoughts as well as specific information without concern for the consultant's judgment or rejection. An example of catalytic intervention is the cooperative collection of information so that the consultee may achieve a clearer statement of the problem and possible solutions. Confrontational interventions challenge the consultee to examine the present thinking or perceptions and are aimed at providing a more accurate picture of the situation. A consultant may tell the consultee what to do (give a prescription) in order to resolve a situation. In this situation the consultant assumes responsibility for formulating the resolution and recommending the specific action. Finally, the consultant may teach theories or principles that are important to the problem so the consultee can learn tested ways of learning the situation and rectifying it. A consultant may use one form of intervention exclusively; however, most will use several types of interventions in each consultation situation.

Determining Course of Action

The particular steps of the intervention are outlined and a timeline set for completion. Returning to the contract to determine who will be responsible for what action may prove helpful. Setting up a period of strategy review will provide feedback later on and will work to reduce resistance. If a strategy is looked upon as a trial run, consultees may be more willing to try it out and participate in an evaluation of its effectiveness (Walz and Benjamin, 1978).

Determining the course of action will again require a review of the impacting variables such as physical, personnel, and financial resources. There may be others which are less explicit; for example, there may be political ramifications or the cultural or standardized norms of the consultee (individual, group, or organization). The more awareness as to what these variables are, the more likely that any suggestions for options made by the consultant will not be rejected by the consultee.

If one follows the process model of consultation, one of the goals will be to increase the effectiveness of the consultee to engage in problem-solving behaviors in the future. It would then be important to design interventions which do not increase or maintain the dependency on the consultant, but assist the consultee in developing feelings of competency to do problem solving. In this manner, collaborative consultation can be empowering for the consultee.

There are both consultee and consultant variables to consider in this phase. Questions to be asked include: Does the consultee or consultant possess the necessary skills to implement the plan? How does the gender, race, or socioeconomic condition of the consultee or consultant affect the acceptance of influence of the other? What is the commitment and motivation to change at differing levels and at this stage in the process? What are the values and ethics of the parties involved? These are all issues of assessment which need clarification when determining intervention.

One factor in selecting an intervention is the decision to work with individuals or groups. Often in working with organizations consultants believe it is important to use team approaches, particularly in problem solving that will affect the larger organization. However, Casey and Critchley (1984) found that the experiencing of trust and openness in team discussions is desirable but not always necessary for successful decision making. They conducted a case study to examine decision making and found that about 10 percent of decisions made by managers could be classified as strategic to the future success of the whole organization and, therefore, requiring the top management to share ideas and feelings equally. Ninety percent of the decisions were more operational and made by individuals, groups, or departments, and were based on specific goals, data, and expertise. Casey and Critchley suggested that decision-making work groups were helpful when there was more uncertainty and, therefore, a need to share. Since difficult decisions create uncertainties, these may require the sharing of each individual's ideas and feelings.

Another consideration in selecting an intervention involves the timing in which the consultant is contacted. Kurpius (1985) points out that work groups and sometimes whole organizations tend to pass through developmental phases and that recognizing these phases can be beneficial for the consultant. He identified four commonly observed phases: (1) development, (2) maintenance, (3) decline, and (4) crisis. With each phase there are different norms, feelings, and behaviors. During the early development of a program there will be different ideas and concepts about the goals and how to proceed. Although staff members are highly motivated, differences of opinion provide potential conflict. Later, the members will have established a clearer understanding of the task and be more goal directed, and they can focus on both the task and the relationship. Therefore the consultant's interventions, which help with goal and role clarity as well as conflict resolution, will be helpful during this phase. Establishing a relationship and improving teamwork are important as they move into the maintenance phase. During the early maintenance period the members are enjoying some of the stabilization of the program which has resulted from the conflict resolution and hard work. However, after a period of time, some people feel a need for additional change while others will be satisfied with the present situation. Because the various points of view are often relatively balanced at this time, turf-protection behaviors may emerge, and eventually competitive behaviors may be observed in the different camps. It is clear that the consultant will need to reinstitute the relationship-oriented interventions as well as conflict resolution procedures during this period. However, survey feedback and some staff training may help them to clarify goals and establish priorities and processes to reach them. The period of decline in an organization occurs when the staff has been trying to resolve issues on its own and now recognizes that change will not be possible without outside assistance. In fact, this is the most frequent time that consultants are sought. When consultants enter an organization at this time, they are going to be encountering the turf-protection and competiton between the different points of view. There may be a surface level of cohesiveness among the members because they do want a resolution. However, when the real work begins, the separate factions may display their anger—the defensiveness and turf-protection surfacing. Obviously, it is necessary for members to return to the development phase. Planned or natural staff changes may modify some of the resisting forces and add some new ideas. The consultant's role is to move the decision making back through the development stage and into a period of maintenance.

There are times when an agency does not ask for help or when a consultation is not successful in helping the group recycle. In such a situation the work environment continues to decline and a crisis may occur. The early stage of crisis involves much denial, and outside forces are resisted while high stress and low productivity occur among the work force. This atmosphere may continue with little hope of recovery unless there is as restructuring or reorganization. Usually some type of outside control takes over and restructuring and reassignment begins to occur. If this continues, the early development behaviors will begin and the system will move through the creative formulations of program development.

In her study, Lovelady (1984) reported that consultants tended to offer vague, unformed reasons as to why they had chosen certain methods. They could describe what had occurred on the project but rarely explained why they had chosen particular methods. She was able, however, to glean the criteria of selection from consultants' descriptions and reported the most commonly used. One reason for selecting an intervention was that the consultant already had the skills needed. The consultant had used the data-gathering method or other consulting intervention previously and felt comfortable with it. Another criterion was to respond to the consultee's expectations as the consultant perceived them. At times the consultee or organization has its own ideas of what it needs and emphasizes its own choice of intervention. Cost, both in money and resources, is another reason for a consultant using a particular intervention. Having workshops conducted for staff members on-site is less expensive and keeps employees at the workplace. Most difficult to define was impact of organizational culture and norms of behavior. However, there was evidence from the consultants in the study that some more or less specific estimate of the culture does occur. These listed criteria suggest that the matching of interventions to demands is a complex process and one which is highly situationally determined. It also indicates that consultants work with rudimentary frameworks in selecting interventions.

Implementation

Implementing the plan can involve various procedures and techniques depending on the level of intervention, time constraints, goals, money, level of risk or change required, and the consultee/consultant individual variables. The purpose of implementation is problem solving, and to initiate and maintain problem-solving behaviors in the consultee. Techniques include but are not limited to: role playing, modeling, positive reinforcement, didactic experiences, providing feedback, mediation, group cohesive activities, and group sessions.

In the expert model, when the consultant is called upon to provide information about a specific problem, she may find skill and knowledge deficits on the part of the consultee, which suggests some educational and developmental activities in conjunction with recommendations. In a systems context, the process model—where there is greater collaboration and the goal of increasing the effectiveness of the consultee—more sophisticated techniques found in the theoretical bases of cognitive restructuring or cognitive-behavioral frameworks may be appropriate. Regardless of the intervention decided on, there must be agreement of the parties involved.

Beer (1980) proposed a set of rules in making decisions about integrating organizational interventions. These rules also seem appropriate for most consultation situations. When the consultant is not knowledgeable of the situation, interventions that maximize the diagnostic information should be used first. The consultant should then order interventions in a manner that maximizes their effectiveness. The consultant should order interventions to better use the organizational resources such as time, money, and energy. And, intervention should be ordered to maximize speed to attain organizational goals. Interventions should be selected that are most relevant to organizational needs and that minimize psychological and organizational strain while insuring individual confidence and commitment to organizational improvement.

Lovelady (1984) outlines intervention methods which are used for organizational development consultation. The general outline is also appropriate for most consultation activities. The following interventions are grouped into activities intended to achieve a similar purpose.

A. Planning Activities
    1. Gap Theory—Data collection and discussion of the current state and the desired future state.
    2. Alternative Futures—Group discussion of possible alternatives and consequences of each.
    3. Systems Modeling—Using data to model a picture of the current situation including the interactions of the system and then using it to trace the consequences of the changes in the system.
    4. Open Systems Planning—Using an open systems framework to identify key aspects of the system and system interactions to plan and monitor changes.
    5. Structural Analysis—Analyzing roles, responsibilities, and communications in the structure.
B. Problem-Solving Activities
    1. Small Group Problem Solving—Mixed groups according to discipline or level working together on the solution or a task with the assistance of a consultant.
C. Learning Activities
    1. Training Activities—Job training, technique training, knowledge training. The training may be conducted by an expert rather than the consultant.

    2. Training and Interactive Skills—Presentation skills, appraisal skills.
    3. Training in Group Interaction—This would include a range of techniques such as t-groups.
D. Process Activities
    1. Process Consultation—Methods used to assist in the process of interaction and to enable activities to take place more efficiently in groups.
E. Role-Centered Activities
    1. Role Clarification and Analysis—Using a structure or framework to clarify individual and group roles.
    2. Role Negotiation—Between individuals and positions.
    3. Group-dynamic Exercises—Examine the roles played in the group by individual members.
F. Task, plus Learning Activities
    1. Residential Courses and Away Days—Taking a group of employees out of the work environment to spend time learning, planning, and working together with subobjectives of improving communication and interaction.
G. Individual Activities
    1. Counseling Activities—Working on a one-to-one basis to help an individual with personal or interpersonal problems or to give personal support.
H. Structural Change Activities
    1. Structural Changes—Redefinition of jobs and responsibilities, reexamining of levels in the structure and the relationship between functions.
I. Action
    1. Making Changes—A broadly defined category that describes the vast array of changes which the consultant and consultee agreed upon.

TERMINATION

Consultations may terminate after the selection of an intervention, leaving the consultee to carry out the plan and evaluate it. In most situations, however, the consultant is involved in the process as the consultee implements the intervention and then both are involved in the evaluation.

Evaluation

Evaluation may be a continuing part of the process of consultation but certainly should be involved prior to termination. Brown, Kurpius, and Morris (1988) suggest that all too often evaluation is avoided or planned in a haphazard manner. This may occur because evaluation and research are confused. Research is designed to add to a field's knowledge base or to support a theory by predicting outcomes or explaining relationships between or among different variables. Evaluation focuses on a single setting and its consultee and client system (Gallessich, 1982). An evaluation can provide meaningful information about the consultant's role, consultee changes, and the impact of the changes on the system. Evaluations are used in making decisions about continuing services, modifying interventions, or that progress has been satisfactory. Data from an evaluation will serve as a guide for the consultant not only in this particular situation but also in developing future consultation projects. Evaluation confirms for the consultee that changes have taken place to a satisfactory degree.

It is important that the evaluation involves consultant's and consultee's behavior as well as the effects on the client or organization. If the evaluation of the consultation is positive, the consultee must decide whether continuation of the consultation is necessary and, if so, how that would be accomplished. If the consultation outcome is negative, the consultant and consultee need to determine if the lack of success is due to ineffective procedures or personnel resistance. They must also determine whether that approach should be altered or a new plan chosen and, if necessary, repeat the steps for the procedure selection. Redmon and colleagues (1985) suggest that the evaluation phase at least should include an interpretation of the data collected after the change has been implemented, continue the current plan if it is supported, or recycle and return to earlier stages if it is not, and avoid premature changes. They also note that the consultant should not take sole responsibility for either success or failure.

Some reasons for failure.   Clearly consultation does not always succeed. In fact, the research regarding consultation is such that it is difficult to determine the rate of success. It is worthwhile examining some of the factors that contribute to failure so that future consultations can consider these variables in the planning stages and hopefully avoid them. Kurpius (1985) provides an excellent overview of some common reasons for failure in consultation. He believes some consultants set impossibly high goals and often link those with the improper intervention. McClelland (1978) reported that many social-change goals are unachievable and that the technology applied is also inappropriate and owned primarily by interventionists. McClelland labeled these "power goals" because the decision makers appear to be more interested in making an impact on others around them than accomplishing something for those in need. Weick (1984) reported that "people often defined social problems in ways that overwhelmed their ability to do anything about them" (p. 40). When problems are defined in such magnitude, individuals lose interest because the problems seem unsolvable and only contribute to more frustration and helplessness. Weick suggests a process of "small wins," that is, reducing large problems into smaller or understandable, controllable, solvable problems. Solving several smaller problems will establish a successful pattern, thereby reducing the stress and increase interest in participating in subsequent proposals.

Another contribution to failure involves too much or too little assessment. Levinson (1983) believes that consultant self-assessment is as important as consultee–client assessment. The consultant and consultee must be aware of each other's assumptions and the rationale they use for selecting any particular intervention. They must also recognize that the diagnostic process is an intervention in itself. Thus, too much diagnosis can contribute to failure. When data are gathered and not shared with the staff or never used in making a decision, it will contribute to staff dissatisfaction. When an assessment is conducted, people believe that an intervention will be forthcoming. Not only is some change expected, but they hope it will be the kind they want. When those changes do not satisfy them it may contribute to increased stress rather than a problem resolution.

To avoid failure in consultation, some suggest using a systems perspective rather than looking at consultation as a separate entity. Iscoe and Harris (1984) reported that treating consultation and education programs in community mental health centers as separate entities when they had interrelationships was a weakness and stressed the importance of a systems concept to reduce the pattern of independence. Similarly, Adler (1982) suggested going beyond the single approach and toward a larger system of programming in which the whole community was viewed as the unit of analysis. The consultant and consultee need to consider environmental factors within and outside the organization when they are designing interventions, thus emphasizing the importance of the interrelatedness of the systems and broadly defining the unit of analysis. Artise (1984) suggested that interventions occur in a work context and are influenced by the managers instrumental in shaping that work environment. When consultants do not help managers focus on the human interaction, they will contribute to intervention failure.

Maintenance

If the intervention proves successful and the consultee agrees, the procedure should continue and maintenance should be programmed. An intervention that is successful when the consultant is involved may not survive when the consultant withdraws. Therefore, during the maintenance period the responsibility for supervision of the intervention should be transferred to an in-house supervisor. Procedures for collection and review of data on a regular basis need to be established. The person selected to continue in the consultant's role can be based on the roles that were initially designed in carrying out the intervention. When a suitable supervisor has been chosen, procedures for monitoring can be established and the type of data presented and frequency of meetings and methods for changing procedures, when indicated, can be established.

Withdrawal

Beisser and Green (1972) discussed some of the problems encountered in terminating consultation. When the consultant does not allow adequate time for closure, the process may not come to a full and natural conclusion. The consultee may feel left with many problems explored but few decisions reached that they can handle more effectively. On the other hand, personal gratification may be the motive when a consultant or consultee prolong the consultation beyond the time when it is productive in solving the problems. A different problem happens when a consultant assumes the role of a supervisor and appears to evaluate or direct the consultee's or client's work and hold them accountable for their performance.

Schein (1969) described a process of disengagement characterized by three features: a reduced involvement is agreed upon by both consultant and consultee, involvement continues on a very low level, and the possibility of further consultation is made clear. A consultant typically begins withdrawing by decreasing physical presence and using more indirect contact such as the telephone, ultimately leading to all contact being withdrawn. During the maintenance period the consultant is usually available on an intermittent basis to monitor the program. Problems that arise during this time are referred back to the in-house supervisor, and the consultant provides general support to that person. It is important that the consultant avoid premature withdrawal. At times a consultant may leave an organization before it has naturally established conditions to support the program. To avoid this, the consultant establishes criteria for independence on the part of the staff, observing the efficiency with which the program is carried out as the he/she enters the withdrawal process. If all tasks are completed in a timely and efficient manner, the consultant's presence can be reduced to a minimum, until totally withdrawn.

SUMMARY

There are numerous consultation models with a great deal of information which could confuse a consultant without a basic set of procedures. However, most consultation procedures follow a similar set of stages. This chapter presented the stages of consultation. The consultant's conceptualization of problems and training are important in the process. The discussion of initial contact provides guidelines in assessing readiness for change, establishing a working relationship, and developing an understanding of the consultee's situation. A major stage in the process involves assessment and diagnosis. These procedures include gathering data, helping the consultee diagnose, and setting goals to work toward. The intervention stage includes identifying options, determining a course of action, and implementing the intervention to solve the problem. Termination may occur after selection of the intervention, with the consultee doing the implementing, or after the consultant has assisted with the implementation and evaluation of the impact. The process and procedures presented in this chapter will be demonstrated in many of the following chapters.

REFERENCES

ADLER, P. T. (1982). An analysis of the concept of competence in individuals and social systems. *Community Mental Health Journal, 18,* 34–45.

ARGYRIS, C. (1970). *Interventions, theory and method: A behavioral science view.* Reading, MA: Addison-Wesley.

ARTISE, J. (1984). Management development in the United States: A new era in human resource development. Paper presented at World Congress on Management Development, London, England.

BEER, M. (1980). *Organization change and development: A system view.* Glenview, IL: Scott Foresman.

BEISSER, A., and GREEN, R. (1972). *Mental health consultation and education.* Palo Alto, CA: National Press Books.

BERGAN, J. R. (1977). *Behavioral consultation.* Columbus, OH: Charles E. Merrill Publishing Company.

BERGER, N. S. (1979). Beyond testing: A decision-making system for providing school psychological consultation. *Professional Psychology, 6,* 273–277.

BLAKE, R., and MOUTON, J. (1978). Toward a general theory of consultation. *Personnel and Guidance Journal, 56,* 328–330.

BROWN, D., KURPIUS, D., and MORRIS, J. (1988). *Handbook of consultation with individuals and small groups.* Washington, DC: Association for Counselor Education and Supervision.

CAPLAN, G. (1970). *The theory and practice of mental health consultation.* New York: Basic Books.

CARKHUFF, R. R. (1983). *Sources of Human Productivity.* Amherst, MA: Human Resource Development.

CASEY, P., and CRITCHLEY, B. (1984). Second thoughts on team building. Paper presented at Rural Congress on Management Development, London, England.

CHERNISS, C. (1976). Preentry issues in consultation. *American Journal of Community Psychology, 4,* 13–25.

DOUGLAS, J. (1982). A "systems" perspective to behavioral consultation in schools: A personal view. *Bulletin of the British Psychological Society, 35,* 195–197.

DWORKIN, A., and DWORKIN, E. (1975). The conceptual overview of selected consultation models. *American Journal of Community Psychology, 3,* 151–159.

FRENCH, W. L., and BELL, C. H. (1973). *Organization development: Behavioral science interventions for organization improvement.* Englewood Cliffs, NJ: Prentice Hall.

FUQUA, D. R., and NEWMAN, J. L. (1985). Individual consultation. *The Counseling Psychologist, 13,* 390–395.

GALLESSICH, J. (1985). Toward a meta-theory of consultation. *The Counseling Psychologist,* 13, 336–362.

GALLESSICH, J. (1982). *The profession and practice of consultation: A handbook for consultants, trainers of consultants, and consumers of consultant's services.* San Francisco, CA: Jossey-Bass.

GOODSTEIN, L. D. (1978). *Consulting with human service systems.* Redding, MA: Addison-Wesley.

HARRISON, R. (1970). Choosing the depth of organizational intervention. *Journal of Applied Behavioral Science,* 6 (2), 181–202.

ISCOE, I., and HARRIS, L. (1984). Social and Community Intervention. *Annual Reviews of Psychology,* 35, Palo Alto, CA: Annual Reviews.

KOOCHER, G. P., SOURKES, B. M., and KEANE, W. M. (1979). Pediatric oncology consultations: A generalizable model for medical settings. *Professional Psychology,* 8, 467–474.

KURPIUS, D. (1978). Consultation theory and process: An integrated model. *The Personnel and Guidance Journal,* 2, 335–338.

KURPIUS, D. J. (1985). Consultation interventions: Successes, failures, and proposals. *The Counseling Psychologist,* 13, 368–389.

LAMB, H. R., and PETERSON, C. L. (1983). The new community consultation. *Hospital and Community Psychiatry,* 34 (1), 54–59.

LENNOX, N., FLANNAGAN, O., and MEYERS, J. (1979). Organizational consultation to facilitate communication within a school staff. *Psychology in the Schools,* 16 (4), 520–526.

LEVINSON, H. (1983). Intuition versus rationality in organizational diagnosis. *Consultation,* 2, 27–31.

LOVELADY, L. (1984). Change strategies and the use of OD consultants to facilitate change, part 2. *Leadership and Organization Development Journal,* 5, 2–12.

McCLELLAND, D. (1978). Managing motivation to expand human freedom. *American Psychologist,* 3, 201–210.

O'NEILL, P., and TRICKETT, E. (1982). *Community consultation.* San Francisco, CA: Jossey-Bass.

PARSONS, R. D., and MEYERS, J. (1984). *Developing consultation skills.* San Francisco: Jossey-Bass.

PIERSEL, W. C., and GUTKIN, T. B. (1983). Resistance to school-based consultation: A behavioral analysis of the problem. *Psychology in the Schools,* 20, 311–320.

RANDOLPH, D. L. (1985). *Microconsulting: Basic psychological consultation skills for helping professionals.* Johnson City, TN: Institute of Social Sciences & Arts.

RANDOLPH, D. L., and GRAUN, K. (1988). Resistance to consultation: A synthesis for counselor-consultants. *Journal of Counseling and Development,* 67 (3), 182–184.

REDMON, W. K., CULLARI, S., and FARRIS, H. E. (1985). An analysis of some important tasks and phases in consultation. *Journal of Community Psychology,* 13, 375–386.

RUSS, S. W. (1978). Group consultation: Key variables that effect change. *Professional Psychology,* 2, 145–152.

SCHEIN, E. (1978). The role of the consultant: Content expert or process facilitator? *Personnel and Guidance Journal,* 56, 339–343.

SCHEIN, E. (1969). *Process consultation: Its role in organization development.* Reading, MA: Addison-Wesley.

SCHMUCK, R. A., and MILES, M. B. (1971). *Organization development: Behavioral science interventions for organization improvement.* Englewood Cliffs, NJ: Prentice Hall.

WALZ, G. R., and BENJAMIN, L. (1978). A change agent strategy for counselors functioning as consultants. *Personnel and Guidance Journal*, 2, 331–334.
WEICK, K. E. (1984). Small wins. *American Psychologist*, 39, 40–49.
WESTBROOK, F. D., LEONARD, M. M., JOHNSON, F., BOYD, V. S., HUNT, S. M., and McDERMOTT, M. T. (1978). University campus consultation through the formation of collaborative dyads. *Personnel and Guidance Journal*, 2, 359–363.

CHAPTER THREE
CONSULTING
WITH EDUCATIONAL
INSTITUTIONS

Society has undergone changes with which our educational institutions have failed to keep pace. Schools have not adjusted and successfully adapted to the changes evident in society, such as multiculturalism, the changing American family, and population mobility. Fisher (1986) describes communities where the upwardly mobile are characterized by a great deal of competition and schools experience competition which is high. In communities where unemployment is high and the strains of poverty are evident, schools are characterized by autocratic control and a lack of sensitivity for poverty. These are examples of how schools are a microcosm of community life. Because of this, schools are an ideal setting for the work of the consultant.

This chapter will address the need for school consultation and define consultation within educational institutions. We will begin with the understanding of the school as an institution, looking at its unique set of characteristics and its complexity as a system. Stages of consultation within schools will be presented with consideration for the skills and resources needed throughout the process of teacher consultation, parent consultation, administrative consultation, and program consultation. Issues reflecting role conflict, relationships, multicultural influences, resistance, contracting, and ethics will be covered. Models of school consultation and directions for further research will be discussed.

THE SCHOOL AS AN INSTITUTION

The School as a System

The school can be understood as an institution with a unique set of characteristics, yet still resembling a system. It is a system with characteristics of hierarchy, subsystems, and rules. There is a hierarchy, a layering of authority levels within schools, which ranges from the students, who have very little power, to the superintendent, who is seen to have more power than any one group or individual. Schools resemble other institutions and systems, such as the family. The similarity between a traditional family and most schools is no more clearly seen than in the number of males encountered in the hierarchy. As on goes up the ladder of the hierarchy, the number of males increases (Fisher, 1986). The school is a system with characteristic subsystems. These may be groups of teachers, such as departments, department heads, tenured teachers, leaders of the teachers' union, and so forth. Subsystems are formed within the system to facilitate some functional tasks. However, they often serve to hamper other tasks. It is not infrequent that subsystems experience power struggles within the system.

The school is a system with rules. The system's rules strongly influence staff functioning. For example, a school may have the rule that parents are to be held in such esteem that they are not crossed; parents are always appeased no matter what the price. Hierarchy, subsystems, and rules all combine to exemplify how schools are like so many other systems and institutions. At the same time, schools have their own set of characteristics.

The School as a Distinct Institution

The school is distinct as an institution and needs to be appreciated by the consultant who enters the system or, in some cases, is already a part of the system. The outside consultant will need to allow additional time to evaluate the system. The inside consultant, located within the school, will need to step back and gain a more objective perspective of the school. In either case, the consultant will discern the institution in an objective manner. Ideally, schools are most effective in their educational task when there is a good working relationship among the teachers and where mutual trust and cooperation exist. Clear communication among faculty members and other staff facilitates a unified approach to education and one which enhances problem solving. Faculty benefit from a sense of control over the activities in their classrooms and in the school as an institution. Teachers need the ability to link behaviors with problems and understand the association between them. Evaluating problems in this way enables a teacher to prioritize problems which need to be addressed in the classroom. The ability to self-evaluate and accept evaluation also assists a teacher toward appropriate change. Effectiveness in the classroom is increased with the capacity to relate to and work with children with clear, constructive communication, developing a mutual understanding. These healthy characteristics assist in the classroom learning process and ultimately facilitate the process of consultation. When these characteristics do not exist for an individual teacher or for the institution as a whole, the consultant will necessarily be involved in training the faculty.

Problems occur in classrooms when there is a lack of healthy characteristics. Education is limited when problem behavior dominates. Problems occur when, for example, a teacher believes there is little or no control over what takes place in the classroom (Gutkin and Ajchenbaum, 1984). The teacher may often feel there are no solutions available that can institute change. As efforts are made and time goes on with no results, the teacher's perceptions are reinforced and the teacher becomes discouraged. Frequently, problem resolution is attempted by turning the problems over to someone else. It is important for the consultant to understand all of these characteristics as being systemic.

The school consultant needs to assess a school's healthy and unhealthy functioning. This is done at the level of an entire system and also at the level of the individual teacher. The consultation process is many things to a teacher. It may be seen as an easy solution with the consultant being yet another person to whom the teacher can turn over problems. The consultation process usually creates an issue of time for the teacher; it may be viewed as a demand on the teacher's already busy schedule. The rewards to the teacher are often intrinsic and may not be tangible enough for the time and effort. It is likely that the most pressing need for the teacher is to have the problem behaviors brought under control. Gutkin and Ajchenbaum (1984) found the more control teachers feel in dealing with a problem, the more likely they are to prefer consultation rather than referral services. Teachers perceive seeking out and utilizing information as helpful when they have some sense of internal control. The teacher's needs are met when the problem behaviors are addressed and when this allows for an improved learning environment in the classroom. After this is accomplished, the consultant and teacher can begin a longer-term process of building a more rewarding classroom and school climate. When the problem behavior has been addressed, the long-term process can be developed with fewer conflicts in goals. Goal conflict can occur if the consultant has the goal of overall improvement of the school climate and building a rewarding learning environment in the classroom, but the teacher has the more immediate need for correcting or controlling behavior problems. Each goal sought is based on the perception of the individual. Goal conflict can be reduced when the consultant and consultee become partners in a collaborative consulting relationship. The consultant's outside position provides an objective view of the classroom while the teacher's inside perception offers a great deal of information and history about the class system.

Schools are highly complex institutions. Within the setting an organizational flow exists with communication and direction building from principals to teachers to students. Consultants need to be involved with school administration, parents, teachers, and students. Influence in the areas of growth and change can be effected in a comprehensive way by including all participants of the school's system. Power structures exist and are not always the same on informal and formal levels. For example, it is often the case that a formal structure for communication exists between administrators and teachers. This may be in the form of staff meetings, memos, or committee meetings. Whatever the mode, the communication process is formal and is known to all faculty. However, communication is most often transmitted on an informal basis. Everyone inside the organization knows the process for this communication and is accustomed to it. An outside consultant, however, will need to assess the communication style, consciously looking for the method of relating information and associated patterns.

STAGES

Entry and Diagnosis

Entry in the school system is best accomplished at higher levels of the system. Working with the administration facilitates a good working relationship and good communication within the system. Even when the consultant is invited into the consultation process by a teacher or teacher group, the consultant should work with the administration for the purpose of a good working relationship. Consultants need to consider the structure of power in the institution. The formal power structure is not the only existing power. It is also important to determine patterns of authority exhibited in other ways. Assessing power by observing communication patterns, such as the flow of communication, who speaks to whom, and who listens, is very beneficial. The consultant may observe power structures that are surprising. For example, veteran teachers may wield a great deal of authority in a school or, in some cases, the consultant will find that parent or community groups will have a good deal of power. The consultant will also want to assess the system's coping capacities. Each system has adjusted to changes in policy, staff, student population, and community alterations in its own way. These coping strategies may be healthy or unhealthy. They are used, however, because they work. The consultant needs to recognize the strengths of the system and its limitations. The limitations may, in fact, become areas for growth. In addition, the consultant should identify the resources available to the institution as well as the obstacles to success. Evaluation of the school will provide the consultant with an understanding of the problem-solving patterns commonly used by those in the system. The consultant should also have an assessment of the hierarchical levels of the system, identifying who is at each level as well as the rigidity of the levels. This is very important in guiding the consultant in his/her communication since communication typically follows the hierarchical levels within a system, at least on a formal basis.

The entry stage of consultation will also be instrumental in assessment of the multicultural dynamics of the school. The particular process of evaluation used by the consultant should be influenced by an understanding of and appreciation for the dominant cultural background(s) of the school and the school community. Cultural and ethnic characteristics will also influence expectations the consultant will develop for the consultation process. This should be the case regardless of the consultant's own cultural and ethnic background. The consultant needs to acquire an appreciation for and a sensitivity to the school community.

School consultants will have more impact along the various stages of consultation if they have access to high-level school staff. The entry stage of a consultation process is important for obvious reasons. This stage sets the tone of the experience for all involved. The consultant wants to be especially sure of gaining the necessary power to effect change within the already-established system. Access to administration within a building can be helpful because a building principal, for example, will transfer authority to the consultant. Even if a teacher feels positively about the consultant, the sanctioning of the consultant's involvement with teachers by the principal will add the needed authorization. This will promote the efforts of the consultant and reinforce the program of consultation. The consultant will be involved with contracting early in the entry stage of consultation. Contracting is negotiated between the contact person(s), usually the administration, and the consultant. This process is beneficial to both parties because it helps to establish goals and set limits. Contracting makes clear what will and will not be done. Contracting necessitates a process of diagnosis which takes into account the limitations and gifts of the school and its staff. The contract statement is descriptive and informative, offering a clear, objective picture of the situation. The diagnostic statement should take into account what is reasonable to accomplish in the period of time with the given resources. The consultant needs to remember perceptions may differ from that of the consultee. It is also possible that needs may change, which can result in a revised contract. The consultant must always be aware of the communication process; it is important to use diagnostic language that best relates to the consultee(s). The more descriptive and objective, the more useful it will be to those needing to make the changes. A written contract may describe (1) the problem defined, (2) the approach to problem resolution agreed upon by the participants, (3) the consultant's role, (4) the number of meetings or seminars to take place, (5) the intervention approach or strategies, and (6) how the consultation will be evaluated (Fisher, 1986). When the contract is written as a formal letter, it concretizes the agreement and short-circuits potential problems.

Intervention

The stage of intervention requires all the various resources the school administration can offer for an effective consultation program. Administrative support is essential at this stage because it is now that difficult work begins, especially for those administering the intervention strategies. They are usually teachers who, as described previously, are often already overbooked. Support is necessary. The administration can assist by providing additional space for intervention activities to take place, such as for timeout strategies with acting-out children. Space within a school is usually at a premium, so offering room for activities, even for the consultant to meet with the teacher, is an act of affirmation of the program. Time is another valued and difficult-to-find item within schools. It is usually left to the administrator to arrange time for a program. The principal will need to be encouraged by the consultant to free the classroom teacher in such a way that the teacher sees consultation not as an extra burden but as a benefit. The stage of intervention can be viewed as a stage of reality. It is the first time the staff recognizes the full dimension of the concern(s). Because the school is a system, with one level or area impacting on another, any given intervention will necessary impact on other aspects of the functioning of the school. The intervention is expected to create change in a particular way; however, it is often a surprise to find it will create change or need for change in yet another area. Sometimes this surprise is a pleasant one, sometimes it is a problematic one. Multilevel change is productive if the system is ready for it. On the other hand, change may result in resistance and suspicion. This reaction may lead to a redefinition of the consultation contract and perhaps longer-term consultation with the school. Whether or not the school wishes to resolve the sources of resistance and make the needed additional changes, the response to change needs to be addressed in an honest way. The response should be described and the choice for dealing with it should be included in the final report. This brings us to the last stage of consultation, that of evaluation.

Evaluation and Closure

The final stage, evaluation, is one that is planned at the stage of entry. It is part of the contract between the consultant and the consultee. Evaluation adds strength to the consultation program and assists in the direction of any future need for consulting programs. The evaluation process should result in the assessment of the outcome of consultation based on its original goals. The goals must be clear for an evaluation to be useful. Other information than the assessment of goal outcomes may be included in the evaluation. This may be the case when a school experiences change in its system beyond that designed by the original contracted goals of consultation. For example, a school principal may contract with a consultant to train teachers to use behavior change methods in their classrooms. This may involve training time as well as observation time in classrooms. In addition, each teacher will review the intervention strategies and outcomes with the consultant. This program may help faculty appreciate objective observation and encourage interest in further experiences that improve managing the classroom. The faculty may be able to gain from additional time with the consultant, discussing cases and considering approaches beyond those taught in the behavior change module. Or it may be that the administration, who initially set up the consultation for teachers, finds a need for program consultation at the administrative level. These additions would not be reflected in the original goals; however, they need to be addressed in the evaluation, even if they are still in progress and not completed at the time of writing the final report. Also, any goals abandoned for any reason need to be described and the reasons addressed.

Evaluation and outcome documents are often overlooked, especially in institutions that already have a sea of paperwork. The temptation is to negate the importance of writing an evaluation. However, it is part of the consultant's role to see that an evaluation is written, and in a way descriptive of the need for the consultation, the process itself, and the outcome. It is ideal if the evaluation can describe a model which may be used as a guide for future reference in other consultation programs. Consultation outcomes need to be documented. This has been a weakness of programs of this type in the past and one reason why they are not as widely recognized for their benefits as they should be. It is appropriate to briefly include in the evaluation report some of the more significant variables which impact on the outcome of the consultation program. One such variable is that of the culture and ethnic milieu of the school. This provides the setting in which the school exists and in many ways is a backdrop for the rules by which the school functions. Also, the history of the school, its student population, and its personnel are important variables in the outcome of the consultation program. For example, a school history may show that change has not been evident for an extended period of time, in which case it may be resisted. Resistance to change will need to be assessed and the reasons for it respected. Another factor which impacts on the outcome of consultation is the personality of the consultant. The consultant may bring prejudices which impede effective consultation, or may have expectations which are not in line with the needs and/or expectations of the school. Or a consultant may simply not have the ability to interact in a complex system with the varying levels of authority and power. All these areas need to be reflected in the final report.

Closure, the process of termination, is considered early in the entry stage. Closure is not a stage distinct from all other aspects of consultation, to be thought about only when it comes time for the consultant to leave. Termination is a part of the relationship process and should be given care, thought, and planning. In one sense, termination occurs according to the designation in the contract. In another sense, however, termination occurs when the consultee is ready and when the consultant's work is finished. That is, the consultee is functioning independently from the guidance of the consultant, capably handling the issues described at the beginning of the consultation, and working productively and in a healthy atmosphere. Termination is a mutually agreed upon closure between the consultant and the consultee.

Understanding the stages of consultation and how they apply to the school as an institution is important for the management of a good consultation program. Entry, diagnosis, intervention, evaluation, and closure all require consulting skills. The consultant needs to understand the stages as a process whereby each flows into the other. The consultant will do well to understand the institution whether from a position of the inside or outside. The consultant also needs to understand his/her own skills, strengths and limitations. Successful consultation programs are more often those which are contained and focused in a specific area, with defined goals that can best be developed when the consultant knows the institution and his/her own capacities.

ROLE OF CONSULTANT IN TEACHER CONSULTATION

Entry and Diagnosis

A school consultant may consult with teachers from within the system or from outside. When a consultant is already in the system, such as in the role of a school counselor, the consultant has ready access to information on power, communication, history, and other aspects of the school's functioning. The inside consultant does not need to spend time gathering this information. However, the consultant does need to be concerned about objectivity. It may be that the consultant is too close to the situation to accurately evaluate, or it may be that the inside consultant has his/her own agenda. When this is the case, the school counselor should consider not participating in the consultation process. If, however, the choice is to participate under these circumstances, it should be done only with the assistance of supervision, so that the consultant can maintain objectivity needed in the consultation process.

The outside consultant has the responsibility to inform him/herself about the background of the problem, the school, and the dynamics of the structure and the personnel within. The advantage of an outside consultant is objectivity, because there is little or no previous history with the institution. This is very helpful in situations where the problem is intensified by various alignments taking place in the school. The consultant is usually seen as not aligned with anyone, with the possible exception of the association with the contact person(s). The inside consultant lacks this objectivity. However, the inside consultant has the advantage of having information prior to the beginning of consultation; this is a limitation with which the outside consultant has to contend. It is a longer process for the outside consultant at the beginning of consultation when time is spent gathering information which the inside person already has on hand. This time may very well be balanced, however, against the process which takes place following entry. The outside consultant brings an image of the expert to the process which the inside person cannot automatically have among his/her colleagues. This image offers power, so resistance to the consultation program is minimized. People tend to give the role of expert more readily to an outside person than to an inside person, unless it has first been established.

Whether consulting from inside or outside, the consultant needs to be professional in the approach used in all stages of consultation. It is important to develop a relationship of mutual trust and cooperation with the staff in the entry stage. If this is missed, the program may not succeed. Clear communication is useful in the development of professional relationships. Confidential treatment of all data gathered in the diagnostic stage is essential. School personnel will recognize professional handling of material and will provide material more willingly when they see a consultant respecting confidentiality. Diagnosis which is not only professionally developed but also described for the school staff in clear, descriptive terms is far more useful and goes a long way in building better communication. In addition, this kind of diagnostic work will contribute to the successful outcome of the goals of consultation. Part of the diagnosis is an understanding of whose problem is being addressed. It is important to note that a problem may be described as belonging to one party when in fact it is a problem for another. This is common in a classroom when a teacher notes the out-of-seat behavior of a student. The teacher may discuss this behavior in terms of interference of the student's work; however, it is highly possible the behavior is really not at all a problem of the child. The problem is more a concern of and likely a disruption for, the teacher. The teacher finds the behavior interruptive and objectionable. Therefore, it is a problem of the teacher's, who has identified it as a problem of the child's.

Intervention

Intervention in teacher consultation varies according to the type of problem and is not primarily affected by the origin of the consultant, whether inside or outside. Yet, it remains a difficult and exciting stage for the teacher. The teacher will undoubtedly have mixed feelings about intervention. Intervention brings change, and change, even when desirable, requires adjustment. To introduce change in a classroom means the teacher is taking a risk. Old behavior patterns are substituted for new. When the class clown stops clowning and settles down to work, the class loses its entertainment and the child loses the role which had served to provide much desirable attention. New patterns change all that. New patterns of behavior require time for the child to adjust to a new identity and for the class to adjust to new expectations for the child. The teacher deserves support from the consultant in this risk—yet support without allowing the teacher to "turn over the problem." The teacher will need to hear that resistance is a common response to behavior change and that time along with consistent teacher responses will facilitate a successful outcome. The teacher needs to support the children involved in the changes; however, the consultant needs to support the teacher. The more substantial the support and encouragement received by the teacher from the consultant, the more capable the teacher becomes in offering the same to the children, modeling behavior learned from the consultant.

Evaluation and Closure

Evaluation and closure in teacher consultation needs to address the dynamic of relationship. From the point of entry, the consultant has been concerned with building a relationship with the teacher defined by trust and mutual respect and understanding. This is a relationship unlike that of a counseling relationship. The teacher is recognized as a professional with many skills. The teacher is the critical figure and the key to working with the child's problems. Therefore, if the consultant has succeeded in communicating this message and acquiring the teacher's trust, closure of the consulting relationship requires special attention. The teacher deserves specific feedback about the experience as perceived by the consultant. The teacher will benefit from hearing the consultant's assessment of the teacher's behavior. The consultant needs to leave the teacher with the sense of goal accomplishment and belief in self for future ideas in the classroom. The teacher should conclude the consultation process feeling positive about the experience, feeling independent about new classroom behaviors and perceptions, and with a sense of courage toward new goals.

Case example.   Teacher consultation has been affected by PL 94–142, the Education for All Handicapped Children Act. This law, passed by Congress in 1975, is a response to the public demand for appropriate special education services and the elimination of discriminatory assessment practices. What is established by the Act is a formula for providing financial assistance to states based on the number of handicapped children receiving special education and related services. The provisions of the Act were designed to ensure free and appropriate public education to handicapped children and their parents, and to ensure the effectiveness of special education programs for the handicapped. Teacher consultation is a common approach in assisting teachers who are working with handicapped children in mainstreaming. Mainstreaming is affected by the regular classroom teacher, who is trying to integrate a handicapped child and implement provisions of the child's educational plan. The following case of Anne demonstrates a teacher consultation role in this kind of situation.

Anne is an 11-year old Learning Disabled student who was placed in a resource room and mainstreamed for math, science, social studies, art, gym, and music at the fifth-grade level. Anne's Individual Educational Plan (IEP) mandates the mainstreaming and other modifications, such as audiotaped instructional materials to facilitate her lessons in reading since she is slower than the other students in the fifth-grade class. The IEP is specific and clear about Anne's needs for which the teacher is responsible. The teacher is the consultee needing assistance in handling this new situation.

The consultant functions as a resource person. The teacher needs assistance in acquiring information necessary for teaching Anne, such as texts and recording services. Until now, the teacher has been able to approach all children with similar materials and a common teaching style, so teaching Anne is overwhelming for the teacher. The teacher must sort feelings of inadequacy and confusion. The consultant can provide materials and ideas for the teacher. In addition, the consultant functions as a facilitator. The consultant is able to encourage cooperation in the teacher, and between parents and school personnel. Clear communication between the people involved in Anne's education promotes consistency in her program and facilitates decisions made. For example, it is important to select the right time to challenge Anne in her academic work. It is also helpful to know when to allow time without direct challenges. All decisions are important enough to make carefully and with the consideration of the people involved in Anne's life. For example, the decision for placement in the following school year is a more complex decision than with other children. The regular classroom teacher has little time for the necessary coordination of Anne's program and the decisions to be made. Since it is important that one person remain in touch with all involved with and concerned about Ann's well-being, it is reasonable that a school consultant should take this role.

Two people who need to communicate are the special education teacher involved in designing Anne's IEP and the regular classroom teacher carrying out the instructions of the IEP. These two people remain actively involved with Anne but in entirely different settings; their goals are the same, yet they approach them separately. It becomes important for the consultant to keep these two people connected and communicating. The consultant will be the liaison between them. Their individual observations of and concerns for Anne provide a more complete picture of Anne's progress.

The consultant is free to move between the settings in which Anne works. The consultant can monitor these settings and assist with questions and concerns raised by the individuals involved. It is not unlikely that the regular teacher will express reluctance or even annoyance regarding Anne's placement because of the implications for the teacher and the classroom. The teacher may ask some legitimate questions in an attempt to understand and accept Anne and the IEP stipulations: "Do I have the skills necessary to teach Anne?" "What effect will Anne have on other students?" "Should I prepare other students for Anne's entrance?" "How do I discipline her?" "Do I use the same grading standards for Anne as the other children?" "This makes twenty-eight students in my class, but doesn't the special ed. teacher have only ten plus the help of an aide?" These questions are important and the consultant should be ready to help raise and explore them. At the same time, the consultant can offer support to the teacher. The consultant can use the model of consultee-centered consultation in working with these issues and questions of the teacher. In this way the focus shifts from the client to the teacher's concerns. The consultant provides a setting and environment to process the inner feelings of inadequacy felt by the teacher in dealing with Anne as well as the anger and jealousy for the special education teacher.

It may be necessary to clarify the consultation goals and the role of the consultant during this period of intervention. The consultant can define the goal: The goal is the success of mainstreaming Anne and *not* to supervise the teacher. This may relieve the teacher from feeling on the spot.

Also, emphasizing the collaborative nature of the role is important to the success of the consultation. All questions need to be addressed and possible resolutions discussed. For example, if class size is a continuing issue for the regular classroom teacher, the consultant may explore the possibility of the special education teacher working with some of the students in the regular classroom as a trade-off.

Finally, the role of consultant in the case of Anne appropriately includes the role of advocate. The consultant is the only person who has perspective on Anne's overall behavior. The consultant is linked with the parents at home, identifying any behavior change and/or improvement, with the special education teacher, and with the regular classroom teacher. The breadth of information the consultant has available makes it possible to objectively evaluate Anne's strengths and limitations. The consultant is able to provide continuous monitoring of home–school activities, regular and special staff interactions, and student–school dynamics which give important information regarding Anne's successes and problems. This position permits the consultant to advocate for needs Anne may have, such as determining the best environment in which Anne may learn, given Anne's personality characteristics, those of prospective teachers, and types of learning atmospheres available at school.

The Impact of PL 94–142 on the School Consultant's Role

The consultation role is expanded in the case of a mainstreamed handicapped child, especially for the inside consultant who may have the role of school psychologist. The consultant can appropriately act as facilitator for the educational program, linking with all the important parties in the child's life. The consultant is able to advocate for the best possible alternatives for the child. The consultant can teach the regular classroom teacher ways of incorporating a handicapped child in the classroom. Then, the next time a child with special needs is included in the class, these will be skills the teacher will already have. Thus, the consultant is available for assistance to all parties, within the parameters of the goals for mainstreaming the child.

Consultation in school is affected by the Education for All Handicapped Children Act, and the act has conflicting implications. It puts greater numbers of handicapped children in regular programs, meaning the teachers working with these children have greater need for consulting services. The teachers face children who they feel ill prepared to teach. Unfortunately, no consulting role has been written into the legislation. The trend has been to place greater emphasis on individual psychoeducational diagnostic procedures (Berger, 1979; Alpert and Trachtman, 1980; and

Fairchild, 1982). This approach is costly and time consuming. As the trend for mainstreaming has developed, however, the need for teacher consultation has increased.

PL 94–142 requires that choices be made by the school consultant in conjunction with the administration. The consultant's role needs to be evaluated in light of the various demands of this act and its impacts. Choices need to be made regarding expenditures of time. The consultant is asked to determine how the law will be interpreted and implemented. Many chose to increase time allotted to psychoeducational assessment. This is a correct interpretation but impacts on the role of consultant. The effect may be so strong that consultation may be "sentenced to the death penalty" (Alpert and Trachtman, 1980), especially with those in the role of school psychologist. The consultant who spends much of his/her time in assessment has little or no time left for consulting work with teachers, parents, or administrators. It is an issue of direct versus indirect services. However, one cannot exist without the other without there being a cost to some part of the program. Indirect service which involves mental health consultation is needed by teachers, parents, team members, and the institution. The consultant needs to have the vision to broaden the traditional role and develop a comprehensive teacher-consultation approach.

THE ROLE OF THE SCHOOL CONSULTANT IN PARENT CONSULTATION

Parent consultation is an appropriate aspect of the school consultant's role. Many parents are very interested in their children's educational progress and may seek out the help of a consultant. They are, at least, very likely to be responsive to the initiations of a school consultant when contacted about their children. Other parents are more fearful and suspicious of schools, teachers, education and, consequently, school consultants. This is frequently true because they have had few, if any, positive experiences with schools and school personnel. It may seem that these are the people with whom consultants most often find themselves working. Whether or not this is actually the case, the resistance stemming from suspicion and fear is a sign of the parents' needs in consultation. It becomes very useful for the consultant to have an understanding of family dynamics. Family work is described in another chapter, so for now it is worth noting only as an area the school consultant may explore for increased understanding of parents.

Parent consultation is very useful in conjunction with teacher consultation. Parents represent the other major part of the world of children. There are opportunities for the parents to oversee assignments at home, to provide a reasonable atmosphere for studying, to provide encouragement, to be involved in contracts between the teacher and the student, to be a part of the reward system, and to provide feedback regarding the child's behavior at home. There are many benefits to the child's general progress that only the parents can offer. This permits a collaborative approach in working with parents—respecting their position and their role with their children.

Contact with parents is also possible without previous connection with the teacher. The parents may initiate this contact out of their own concern. Since parents now have more rights—access to student records, organizations that emphasize parental involvement—increased parental involvement is likely to result in more parental initiation. Parents who initiate contact with the school need a connecting person, a liaison. The school consultant is able to participate in this role. For example, when parents who want to inspect school records contact the school, the school consultant can be available to offer an interpretation of the records. Teacher comments and test scores can be described in context with the wider picture of the child's experience. Parents who know someone will respond positively to their inquiries and assist them in their questions will more than likely return to the school with a favorable attitude and will be able to consider a collaborative role with the school in the future.

Case Example

Parent contact by the school consultant is entirely appropriate and, in many circumstances, necessary for the benefit of children. This is demonstrated in the case which follows. Mark is a six-year-old student who has been labeled as educationally Multiply-Handicapped. He has severe speech and language delay; is very active; shows a discrepancy between verbal and performance abilities; and it is suspected that test scores are deflated due to emotional factors. Mark has made little progress academically and behaviorally. The classroom teacher asked the consultant to help identify possible reasons for the lack of progress. In response, the consultant contacted school personnel who were individually involved with Mark, such as the speech therapist, reading specialist, and physical education teacher. They met together with the classroom teacher and the consultant to discuss diagnostic issues and remediation possibilities. It was decided the parents needed to be contacted because of the extent of Mark's behavior.

Entry and diagnosis.   Consultation regarding Mark had already started by the time the parents were contacted. However, it was necessary for the consultant to view the introduction of the parents to the process as a new beginning. It was another entry level stage, now, with the parents present. The consultant was the contact person and would remain as liaison for all involved in Mark's case. The consultant invited the parents to contact her at any time. It was important to remember the reluctance the parents were likely to have. In this case, the parents were hesitant because of Mark's lack of progress. They were not surprised at the contact, but were ambivalent and anxious. The consultant was careful to make the first interview one characterized by listening, problem solving, and minimizing defensiveness. Any reference to negativity between Mark and his parents was reframed by the consultant. For example, the parents, who had had no success in dealing with Mark at home, presented many of their problems. Often they blamed Mark for his inappropriate behavior. They complained because Mark would go off to play without telling them or would try to do things he saw others doing and become frustrated. The parents reported that it was useless to try to talk to him. The consultant reframed many of these incidents in ways which explained reasons for Mark's behavior. At times the reasons were as simple as his age. The consultant explained in developmental terms what a nonhandicapped six-year-old child could be expected to accomplish. Other times Mark's behavior could be explained by his handicaps. It was important for the consultant to provide careful descriptions which offered clarity. Examples were used to present a complete picture of the situation. Many of these examples were from the classroom, which helped to defuse the parent's defensiveness and assist them in realizing they were not alone in their difficulties with Mark. Information was made available to the parents and terminology was explained. The consultant maintained a collaborative climate, encouraging parental input and problem resolution. The consultant also described the roles of others included in Mark's case. The parents were to be involved with the school personnel as part of a team addressing the needs of Mark. In addition, the consultant would meet with the parents to discuss their ongoing involvement and any questions which they might have. This would permit the parents time alone with the consultant, should they need or wish to discuss family issues.

The parents, teachers, and consultant formed a group to develop a priority list of Mark's needs. They investigated the need for further diagnostic testing, the need for change of placement, and the need for support services such as parent training and family/individual counseling. The consultant assessed the family's motivation and ability to commit to an action plan for change. The consultant also developed a communication network between home and school focusing on Mark's needs. This approach necessitated as much diagnostic work with Mark's parents as with Mark. Time with the parents was important in understanding the meaning of Mark's problems, and this contributed to the diagnostic work.

Intervention.   Implementation of the action plan involved all school participants and the parents at home. It was the responsibility of the consultant to stay connected with the parents during this stage of intervention. The parents needed the support of the consultant and often needed her to clarify goals and the steps to be taken. When discouraged or annoyed with the process, the consultant was able to intervene with the family and assist them in refocusing. The consultant was in an ideal position to guide the family as well as observe the work of the teacher in the classroom and offer support and ideas to both. The climate remained collaborative: the two groups learned from each other and shared ideas. The consultant was conscious the role of collaborator would facilitate such interaction and maintained this approach throughout the consultation. At the same time the consultant acted as evaluator. Keeping enough distance to provide objective observations and by receiving feedback from the parents and teacher, the consultant was able to offer evaluations of what was taking place. The role of evaluator allowed the consultant the opportunity to recommend ongoing changes important for Mark's progress. When negotiations were needed, the consultant was there to initiate them. The consultant remained the pivotal person and the connecting agent offering support and directing relationships.

Evaluation and closure.   The timing of closure was determined by the ongoing evaluation the consultant was conducting. This evaluation process was used to assess the most appropriate time for termination. The consultant wanted to be present as long as the parents were in need of a connecting person; however, the consultant did not want to overestimate her need to stay. The consultant slowly eased out of the role as liaison. Knowing when to leave was determined by how well the parents were able to handle Mark at home and by their willingness to communicate with the teacher on their own. Termination was timely once the parents and teacher had established a working relationship and no longer needed the consultant as go-between and once parent–child relationships were healthy. When this happened, the positive relating between Mark and his parents provided for further positive changes. If this improved relationship does not occur within the normal time of parent consultation, however, the consultant should use her position to refer the family to counseling. Closure with the family may very well occur with the family seeking treatment as a family.

Parent consultation requires an appreciation of the impact a family can have on the child's school behavior. It necessitates an ability to collaborate with parents, respecting what they may bring to helping the child and respecting what they cannot bring. It often requires increased organization and scheduling for the consultant to see the parents. Sensitivity and a delicate sense of timing on the part of the consultant can result in cooperation by the parents—who can be a powerful resource in assisting the client.

THE ROLE OF THE SCHOOL CONSULTANT
IN ADMINISTRATIVE CONSULTATION

Consulting for school administration often involves goals for the total school. When a consultant works with an administrator, an entire faculty may be the concern or, as is sometimes the case, an entire program. The program may be one aspect of the school or it may include all its activities. This often depends on the size of the school.

Crisis resolution may be the model of the consultation. A crisis resolution model does not preclude another approach; however, it may trigger the outside consultant's introduction to the school or the invitation for the inside consultant. A consultant will want to be prepared to look beyond the crisis. It is clear the administration is most concerned with the issue at hand, yet the consultant needs to be oriented toward helping beyond the moment of initial trouble.

The school consultant approaches administrative concerns with the perspective of the systems model. The systems model offers an overview of the institution with its many subsystems all impacting on each other. Consultants oriented to system relationships offer a preventive approach to their consultation. The systems approach permits the consultant to analyze the impact one group has on another and understand the dynamics of the total system—at times, predicting what may be needed for the health of the total system. Thus, the systems approach can offer an expansive view, a preventive one at the optimum. The consultant can also view conflict resolution by understanding the entire system and recognizing the conflict as an aspect of the system's dynamics. For example, classroom problems which typically result in a high number of students being sent to the office for discipline by the principal may not represent teacher inability to handle classroom conflicts. They may, in fact, be an attempt to solicit administrative involvement. Teachers may feel abandoned by the administration, and this may be their not-so-subtle way of receiving assistance and support. The method of handling classroom conflicts is indicative of what is lacking for the teachers. It reveals at least part of the dynamics of the institution.

Collaborative procedures can be used by the consultant which will reach the entire school population and at the same time achieve some of the administrative goals. Collaboration is a key factor in any consultation relationship and is particularly important in administrative consultation.

Trust is most likely to develop in this type of relationship. People can respect one another's positions and maintain objective perspectives which will lead to clear goal definition. Collaborative procedures may be used to achieve goals, such as higher test scores or reduced disciplinary problems. Other administrative goals include problem solving, short- and long-term planning, establishing and maintaining communication channels among teachers and between teachers and administrators, and development of program planning.

Administrative consultation may at times be a component of teacher consultation. When the primary focus of consulting is with teachers, a wise consultant will connect with and, at least informally, consult with the administrator(s). The work of teacher consultation is often enhanced with added consulting with the administration. This is especially the case when, for example, teacher improvement is not clearly supported by the administration. Administrators who lack skills are less likely to encourage teachers to develop skills. Administrators who do not understand the components of effective teaching may not reinforce teachers who can document their effectiveness. Administrators who do not support, encourage, and challenge their teachers may find that teachers lack motivation to perform. Thus, the problems of administrators and teachers are interrelated. This interrelating needs to be recognized by the consultant.

PROGRAM CONSULTATION

A common approach to administrative consultation is program consulting. Program consulting addresses the needs of the institution by focusing on the program rather than on an individual or group. This model is a more complex version of consulting with individuals. It is more expansive and comprehensive. For this reason it is frequently used with administrators who wish to address needs of the institution on a broad scale. The stages of program consultation are similar to those of individual consultation, and many of the issues of consultation are parallel. However, many consultants do not consider this approach because of its complexity. It may seem awesome for a consultant to approach a school on such a comprehensive scale, yet it is the comprehensiveness that is attractive and beneficial. The task of addressing entire programs and working directly with administrators becomes possible when we break the process down into steps. What follows is a description of program consultation defined in stages. The stages will assist in constructing and clarifying the process. After the description of stages, a case will be presented to offer some specifics regarding the application of this approach.

Entry and Diagnosis

Program consultation is often conducted by the consultant with the administration, usually the principal. The consultant needs to obtain permission from high-level administrators for all program consulting in the school. This permission will likely be automatic if the consultant is inside the system. However, the consultant from the outside whose request has come from the principal must be sure of approval from the higher-level administration. High-level administrators may not relate to the purpose of the consultation and, therefore, will not appreciate or support the program. This risk needs to be recognized, as it may block the program. On the other hand, if the consultant is forewarned, communication with the administration can be broached with this in mind. The consultant may be able to divert an administrator's negative reaction.

It is necessary that the administration be clearly informed regarding the nature and scope of the program. These sanctions must be maintained over the duration of the consultation. It is easy for the consultant to forget these higher levels within the system when the consultant is out of routine contact with them. One way to maintain contact is to schedule regular meetings with administrators. Another method is to make informal visits which provide time to offer information and feedback to the administrator. The best choice of the method for systematic contact with the administrator is one the consultant needs to discern. The administrator may suggest a customary approach, or it could be part of a general contract. The chosen approach will be dependent on observations made by the consultant regarding the methods of communication used in the school, the approachability of the administrator, and the style of the consultant.

The consultant will define the consultation process at the entry level. Often consultees will ask for help without understanding the model of consultation. It is helpful to give brief description of consulting and the role of the consultant, defining the working relationship between consultant and consultee(s). This will likely entail a contract, either written or verbal. A written contract is advised. It need not be extensive or detailed. However, it is useful to name the groups involved in the consultation process, the approximate time frame for consultation, the purpose(s), and the fee, where applicable. It is advisable to list any goals in measurable terms and refer to any evaluation and follow-up program which may be planned. At the time of the construction of the contract, the consultant should know all the parties to whom the contract needs to be given. Copies of the contract need to be made available to any who may want to understand the process and/or may want to monitor the program.

Problem identification is an important aspect of the entry and diagnostic stage. The consultant will discover that concern exists for short- and long-term goals. These need to be defined as such with an appreciation for the immediacy of the short-term goals. The consultant will also find lack of clarity of the problem by the various people involved, and/or the problem may be defined differently by them. The described source of the problem may be variant. It is important the consultant recognizes the need to look beyond what is described at the entry level. The consultant needs to listen to others not involved in the initial communication. If the principal is the initiator, the consultant should be prepared to talk with teachers as well. The consultant needs to look at the communication process for patterns which may assist in problem identification. Other areas to pay attention to include methods of teaching, teaching materials, and even expenditures. The consultant needs information regarding goals and specific objectives in areas closely associated with that of the program consultation. These areas may be directly or indirectly impacting on the designated focus for consultation. For example, the focus for consultation is mainstreaming handicapped children into regular classrooms. Yet problems still exist with the introduction of special education classrooms in this particular school. The integration of the special education program has not been complete. The school has some unfinished business and, unless this is attended to, the consulting regarding the mainstreaming program will not be successful. The consultant can be aware of such issues and consider assisting the school in resolving them. Although it may take some extra time at the beginning of the relationship with the school, it can be very helpful. It may also facilitate the intended program.

Short- and long-term goals deserve special attention. The consultant needs to have them clearly defined, as mentioned above. In addition, they can be seen as connected. Short-range goals attend to immediate concerns, long-range goals address the larger issues. For example, a short-term goal may be to reduce inappropriate behavior in the classroom. This is a goal with immediacy because it is a problem obviously affecting many individuals in the school. A long-term goal connected to classroom behavior is selection of new teaching materials. The two are independently important, yet they are connected. Inappropriate classroom behavior may be diagnosed as originating from a level of boredom on the part of the children or, perhaps, the teacher. This makes the selection of new materials an important concern. It is also true that carefully selected teaching materials deserve the consideration of inspired teachers and the best efforts of a "well-behaving" class, if a fair trial period for the material is to be had. The two goals are interconnected.

Program consultation is a dual approach involving human outcomes, such as the reduction of inappropriate classroom behavior, and program outcomes, such as the selection of instructional materials. Both outcomes have their place in consultation. The consultant needs to assist the consultee(s) in distinguishing between these goals and recognizing the importance of each. The danger in not defining each goal is the possibility of premature termination after the first goal has been accomplished. Thus, the consultee may be ready to terminate once only one goal, usually the most frustrating, is met, while the consultant is prepared to continue. The consultant needs to achieve agreement from all involved to move on to the second goal. If a second goal is established after the entry stage, it becomes important to recontract for the second goal. This is best done prior to the accomplishment of the first goal while the consultant is still working with the consultees.

Intervention

The consultant develops a plan of intervention based on problem identification and analysis. The planning process will involve many people who are instrumental to the program goals. They will be individuals who have power to commit resources, influence to lend approval and support, and are responsible for implementation of the intervention plan. Achievement of goals remains the focus. A priority within this goal is the accomplishment of client goals and improvement of the program for the benefit of the clients. This is ultimately the best indication of consultation success.

Many individuals may be actively involved in the program as consultees. This makes the program somewhat complicated. Yet, it should not preclude the consultant's active involvement in maintaining an alliance or relationship with the consultee(s). It is also important to continuously evaluate and clarify the role of all participants so the consultation plan is effectively managed. The consultant should continuously evaluate the contract plan for any needed changes. These need to be fed back to the consultee(s), along with reports on any progress made. Sharing accomplishments offers support and positive feedback to those active in making changes in the system. For intervention to work, all participants need to be clear about the goals, need to feel valued, and need to be connected with others involved in the consultation. Intervention means a lot of consistent work for the consultee(s). The consultant is the key person in making sure the process proceeds smoothly. When consultees do not feel appreciated, they may inadvertently sabotage the process.

Evaluation

Evaluation is an important aspect of consultation. An evaluation process which takes us beyond nondirected, casual conversation can be very informative and has the ability to offer direction for the future. Written evaluations, as contracted at entry, can provide a review of the process of consultation beginning with the inclusion of the personnel involved. The evaluation should also include a description of the goals for consultation, the methods of intervention used, any materials, equipment, or space needed for the program, changes which developed and departed from the original plan, and a discussion of the outcomes. In the discussion of outcomes, a consultant may want to assist the school in future planning and/or future consultations by describing possible directions the school may take as a result of this consultation program's outcomes.

The assessment measures used should be as simple and comprehensive as possible. The simplicity will increase the likelihood of participation by school personnel. If the evaluation technique is too lengthy or complicated, personnel may take a passive approach to the process that will likely result in less than useful responses. Since consultation is a process, the evaluation should reflect this process from beginning to end. It is helpful for the consultant to consider all steps taken to effect the program and design a comprehensive evaluation. One straightforward approach to evaluation is the Likert-type scale, which asks questions specific to the various aspects of the experience. The respondent simply circles the number that best reflects his/her experience. The questions are clear and direct. These can usually be written so that the evaluation is no more than a page in length. There is space provided for additional comments by the respondent. The questions will very likely remind the respondent of the experience and lead to further comments which extend the evaluation material. This results in ratings which can be used in writing the evaluation. These ratings will then allow the consultant to develop some conclusions.

Another form of evaluation is inherent in the intervention process. It is possible to design the intervention so that material is available for evaluation of outcomes. For example, if the consultation is focusing on inappropriate behaviors in a classroom, a baseline can be kept for a given period of time prior to intervention. Then, with intervention clearly marked, the baseline continues showing the change. This can be done with behaviors such as out-of-seat behavior, verbal interruptions, inattentiveness, ignored homework assignments, and shy behaviors. It can also be used when changing teacher behavior, such as overattending to acting-out behaviors, lack of positive reinforcement, administration of poor directions, facial expressions used in teaching, nervousness, and so on. When a baseline is kept faithfully, the data are outcomes which can be used in documenting an evaluation. This is a model that takes more time for everyone involved. The teacher or other personnel need to be trained in making baselines and encouraged in consistent recording. The consultant needs to be involved in this process of training and support. At times, the consultant may have to keep a baseline, for example, on teacher behavior. However, this is an advantage in the long run. Once taught, the teacher can use this approach for outcome evaluations or personal feedback. It is an excellent model and well worth the time of all concerned.

Another model of evaluation is the personal interview. This approach involves the consultant setting up specified interview time with participants. Designated questions are asked of the participants and their answers are recorded. This may be done in a group setting; however, it is best done individually. For this reason, it is a time-consuming process. Moreover, it is often seen as less objective than the other two approaches to evaluation. It is recommended that this type of evaluation be used in conjunction with one of the other models. It can be a useful addition to them; by itself, its comprehensiveness is questionable. An ideal approach to evaluation would be to use all three models described. They are distinct enough to provide a wide selection of data which can be addressed in a comprehensive evaluation report.

The evaluation process needs to receive attention at the entry level of consultation. It is at this time a consultant determines which mode(s) will be used and who will be involved. If the consultant is concerned about evaluation, it would be wise for the consultant to contract for the school personnel to learn models and conduct their own. In some cases, the consultant is time-limited and cannot remain with the school through the end of a comprehensive evaluation. In either circumstance, the consultant may choose that the evaluation work be done by the school. Barbrack (1980) suggests the consultant should know how to conduct a well-designed evaluation but also encourages consultants to train consultees to conduct their own evaluations. Resistance to this process is possible. This may be due to lack of training in the area. The consultant needs to recognize that staff may feel intimidated by the process. Resistance may also be from an unwillingness to review the results. The outcomes may be revealing in an uncomfortable way; they may suggest failure or the need for change. This resistance can be addressed positively and supportively by the consultant.

The written evaluation has the purpose of assessing the outcome of the specified contract goals. The goals need to guide the direction of the evaluation. Other hidden agendas, such as personal vendettas, do not belong. The analysis of the evaluation material can be written in such a way as to highlight the original goals and to reflect possible future directions. When this is done, the evaluation, as well as the consultation program, is of value to the school.

Maintenance and Termination

Maintenance of the consultation outcomes usually occurs over time. The desired changes which have occurred due to consultation need to be maintained, or else they will not be effective. Yet the maintenance program requires additional time beyond the concluding evaluation. This has the potential of creating problems, especially for the consultant. The inside consultant can manage this more realistically than the outside consultant. The outside consultant will need to return to the school for this purpose. An alternative is for the outside consultant to set certain procedures in motion and identify certain people to maintain change which will reduce the consultant's time commitments. In any case, it is important for everyone to recognize that maintenance of change will not occur automatically. Barbrack (1980) indicates it may be more difficult to maintain change than to initiate it. Maintenance of change requires systematic attention and an organized approach. The involvement of the consultees through the consultation program needs to be part of this approach. Once again, this stage needs to be seen as part of a whole process wherein each step is critical to the entire outcome.

Termination is closely connected with the other stages. It comes as a result of the work of the former steps and is part of the contract agreement with the school. Termination needs to be seen as part of the process whereby the consultant and consultee(s) have been in collaboration regarding the goals. Now, when the goals have been met, the evaluation done, and a maintenance program established, the consultant is finished. The consultee experience is one of change and, although the consultation is over, the program will proceed at a new level.

Case Example

Entry and diagnosis. A mental health center interdisciplinary consultation team contracted a program consultation with a local elementary school (Hansen, 1977). The team was made up of psychologists, social workers, teacher consultants, and behavioral technicians. The psychologists, as team leaders, met with the building administrators to develop a contract. This contract was then approved at the higher administration level.

At the entry level, the administrators expressed their concern with the high number of referrals from teachers to school psychologists. The teachers seemed to have difficulty with behaviors in the classroom which the administrators felt should be handled by the teachers. These behaviors included acting-out behavior, such as out-of-seat behavior; excessive noise; and general disruptive behaviors. It was the feeling of the administrators that the teachers could manage more of these behaviors in the classroom.

The consultants diagnosed the stated problems presented by the administration. The teachers were unable and/or unwilling to handle moderate behavior problems. They lacked the knowledge, skills, and the support system to attempt to deal with these problems. Consequently, they referred them out to the school psychologist. Therefore, the teachers' behavior needed to change in order to successfully alter this process. Short-term goals of behavior modification training for the teachers were designed. In order to meet these goals, a six-week training session was developed for twenty teachers who volunteered for the program. This short-term approach was expected to lead to the long-term goal of reduced student referrals.

A schedule of the team's activity in the school was available to the administration. Team members were all introduced at an early meeting and then began the habit of reporting into the school office upon arrival at the school. Consequently, the administrators knew when to expect team members and could connect with them at the times of their arrival and departure. Also, the meeting room was open to all participants at all times, including the administration. The schedule of the team and their accessibility enabled the administrators to remain informed and aware of the activities while retaining a sense of control of the activities in their school. Informal connections which continued throughout the program facilitated the maintenance of administrators' knowledge and support regarding the program.

Intervention. The plan of intervention began when the twenty teachers were given an introduction to the learning theory underlying behavior modification techniques. Two eight-hour in-service sessions were used to present the principles of learning. These focused on observation of student behavior and collection of data. In these sessions, each teacher selected one student with whom the teacher wished to work. The teachers met in small groups with one consultant conducting the group discussion. Each teacher identified the problem behavior and made plans to carefully observe the child and chart the behavior during the week between these two sessions. The teachers were instructed in forming charts for gathering baseline data. The teachers then returned to the second eight-hour session with a week of baseline information regarding the problem behavior.

The next step of intervention was to assist the teachers in developing a workable intervention plan. No intervention strategy had taken place, except the gathering of data based on the teachers' observations. The material presented during the eight hours provided concepts of behavioral change. Small groups were reestablished to process ideas for individual behavioral programs. By the end of the session, the teachers had a plan to begin to alter the child's behavior during the next week.

The consultants met weekly and individually with the teachers for the following four weeks. These meetings were for the purposes of following through on the behavior programs, assuring consistency, answering any questions which might arise in the early weeks of behavioral change, adjusting the program when problems developed, and for teacher reinforcement. In addition, the consultants were preparing the teachers to initiate their second behavioral change plan. The second plan was sometimes established working on yet another behavior of the same child. At times, a second child was selected by the teacher for a new program. In some instances, the teacher chose to work with the entire class using programs which could benefit all the children. These total-class programs were often based on a token economy system of reinforcement. All the new programs were varied and were excellent reinforcement for the teachers' recently learned knowledge. The second experience allowed the material to become a part of the teachers' repertory of good teaching techniques.

The teachers continued their charting throughout the six weeks. In the last session, they shared the outcomes by showing the charted behavior of the child. This approach was a kind of show-and-tell experience designed to reinforce the teachers' behavior. It also showed other teachers some possibilities beyond their own charted outcomes. In some cases the behavior was just beginning to change either because of changes in the program midway or because of the selection of a more complicated behavior which would require a lengthy process of change. By observing one another's cases, the teachers learned a variety of differences in problems, approaches, and children's behaviors.

Evaluation.   Evaluation of this consultation program was inherent in the process. Each teacher was asked to share the baseline chart which was integrated into the final outcome report. In addition, the teachers were given a five-point Likert-type scale for the purpose of written evaluation. The information on this evaluation was also included in the report. A final report was submitted at the conclusion of the six-week program by the consultation team. The report was written by the team with copies sent to building administration, school administrators, and the mental health center. At the end of the semester, after the structured maintenance time period had lapsed, the team used other data to measure the long-term goal: the reduction of student referrals to the school psychologist. Number of referrals for program teachers, and types of referrals, were compared with the nonprogram teachers'. The program teachers had significantly fewer referrals for either active or passive problem behaviors. Short-term and long-term goals were met. In addition, the outcome responses from the written evaluation supported further programs of this type.

Maintenance and termination.   Maintenance of the program was extended beyond the six-week period. When maintenance began, the teacher had accomplished the behavior change strategy of the first plan and was working on a second strategy plan. Maintenance was planned so it would continue with support to the teacher in the various projects. Consultants used an approach of going to the school for maintenance every two weeks for the next two months. This prolonged the time of consultant contact without building dependency on the consultant. It also permitted a reasonable amount of time for termination to be discussed. The experience was one which evolved as part of the process of consultation.

In summary, this program consultation is a good example of a consultation reaching a large number of people and responding to a wide range of needs. Some teachers chose academic issues while others chose to focus on problem behaviors. Teachers varied in their teaching styles. The consultants did not attempt to alter these. The teachers' strengths were assessed and used in developing the intervention approach most suitable to each. Although the program was structured, it was designed to be individualized and adaptable. Dickinson and Adcox (1984) report that a large number of children can be helped in a short period of time by using a consultation program. This suggests a monetary savings for the school. Certain referrals to the school psychologist decrease, freeing that person to respond to other needs. Referral patterns change over time (Hansen, 1977; Ritter, 1978). This happens when referrals are limited to more complex problem behaviors and when a teacher is able to be more specific in describing the referring problem. Teachers who use the consultant in dealing with their students have more collaborative experiences with the consultant. This offers the teachers greater opportunity to develop their own coping skills and approaches. Rather than taking a helpless approach to their problems, they come to know they are quite able to deal with issues they once referred out to someone else. Thus, teachers function more independently and with a greater sense of competency. From year to year, teachers are able to continue to use the training they received. Consequently, many children are able to benefit from this program consultation approach.

Program consultation expands the benefits of individual consultation. Individual consultation is based on the premise that consultation with one teacher provides service to many clients (i.e., the children in that classroom). Program consultation multiplies this by the addition of every teacher to the program. Therefore, a wider mental health and educational service is provided. This means our teachers are better prepared to handle more issues in the classroom and more problems and concerns of the students.

ISSUES FOR THE SCHOOL CONSULTANT

Role Conflict

The role of the internal school consultant is one which means conflict due to the variety of expectations. Conflict exists when many tasks must meet the expectations of the administrator, the teacher, the parent, yet are always performed by the same person, the consultant. The school system is providing services which require altered behaviors on the part of the consultant, such as the complete integration of special education facilities. The administrator must respond to Public Law 92–142, which requires a broader range of services for students affected by the law. Teachers are demanding more assistance with curricular design, behavioral management programs, intervention in crisis situations, individual and group counseling services to students, and in-service training. Parents want information, support groups, and parent education. Methods of evaluation of all programs are being requested. These services typically fall on the shoulders of the school psychologist and school counselor.

Internal and external role conflict exists for the school psychologist. The school psychologist has had the traditional role of diagnostician. This role has come from the psychomedical model in which students are tested, classified, and then placed. The school psychologist's primary role has been testing. Much of this traditional role is being challenged by school staff as well as by the general community. Testing still remains an important aspect of the school program. However, it is no longer the primary demand on the school psychologist's time. This requires a shift for the school psychologist. A broader definition of services delivered has evolved, now including assessment, counseling, staff development, consultation, parent education, liaison, and evaluation. However, major differences still exist for a variety of reasons. Frequently the would-be consultant has been trained only as a psychometrist and chooses to stay in this role rather than expand through professional development and continuing education options. The conflict in this change is often internal. The role is familiar, comfortable, and secure; it is easily defined. The school psychologist is confident in his/her abilities to provide these services. In reality, the caseloads are often so heavy, they consume much time. The paperwork alone leaves little time to provide alternate services. Frequently the school psychologist does not have models to demonstrate alternate approaches. Often, the administrators consider testing to be the only duty of the school psychologist. Lacking vision and a clear understanding of the expanded needs, the administrator frequently supports the limited view and limited role of the school psychologist.

Diagnostic service by practicing school psychologists will continue to be important. However, more responsiveness to consumer needs may be an increasing demand on the school psychologist. This change may be toward assessment and away from testing. Fairchild (1982) describes a service model for assessment consultants wherein assessment consultation is primary and diagnostic assessment is secondary. Good diagnostic skills are not minimized by shifting the emphasis to assessment consultation, since such skills are important to effective assessment. The purpose of this shift is to move responsibilities and more equitably distribute assessment among other school personnel. The assessment consultant selects various assessment instruments and trains people to use tests and interpret them. Often these people are staff who are more intimately involved with the children, such as teachers. They already have developed with the children a relationship which can facilitate a safe testing environment and lead to more accurate test results. This approach recognizes a team approach to assisting a child. The consultant needs to serve as an information synthesizer, pulling all data together for meaningful decision making. The decision making is an effort of a team of people who are connected with the child. The result of this testing approach is a written report which includes the current level of student functioning and specific recommendations. The consultant now has a group of people who understand the process of assessment and, more than likely, appreciate the results. The results of assessment can be applied more effectively when the entire process is understood. This team approach requires a change in attitude on the part of everyone involved. Teamwork necessitates a collaborative atmosphere where all individuals are seen as being able to contribute. Each person has the potential of giving according to one's skills, and each has the capacity of receiving from others on the team. Most important, the client benefits because all team members share the vision of change and collaboration.

Consultants and teachers may realize that children can often be helped in the classroom without administering tests of any kind. Creative assessment models serve more to respect the child's needs than does removing the child from a familiar environment for the purpose of testing. The collaborative approach lends itself to this type of creative model. It reduces the caseload for individual testing and permits more satisfying and comprehensive work when contact with the individual child is necessary. The consultant no longer needs to be the first resort in the assessment process. The team plays this role under the direction of the consultant. Instead of one consultant administering assessments to all children, teams are developed for this purpose. The consultant has an active role in each team, but does not have sole responsibility for assessment.

It is possible to use the traditional direct-service model to define a new and more effective role. Since the direct-service model already exists, it makes sense for professionals to use it to evolve to a more efficient and more encompassing approach which may very well be the model of consultation.

Both internal and external role conflict exist for the school counselor. Typically, the role of the school counselor has not been as clearly defined as that of the school psychologist. The school counselor is often used as a right arm for the administration, which can mean anything from scheduling to discipline. Scheduling is a task which, for many school counselors, falls into the category of clerical work. Discipline directly interferes with the careful relationship-building involved in counseling a child. Yet these variations exist in the counselor's duties, and they lead to conflicts in role.

School counselors who emerge as consultants must struggle in the institution with their image. The history of the school counselor has been one of serving many masters. The school administrator, teachers, parents, and students all have expectations of the counselor's time. The perception of the counselor's role, especially by administrators, often determines the functions they fulfill. This can vary from school to school. One study showed little discrepancy between counselors and administrators regarding the role of the counselor (Bonebrake and Borgers, 1984). Both counselors and administrators ranked teacher consultation and parent consultation high among areas ideally receiving the most emphasis. However, differences were found in disciplinary tasks, supervision, and scheduling. These differences indicate discrepancy in the superficial agreement on consultation. School counselors are handicapped by the lack of a clearly defined job description. Their own image lacks definition. Often they are idealistic about the amount of counseling they would like to do and define their role only as counselor. Frequently, the counselor has moved into the position from the role of teacher and sometimes with sights set toward that of administrator. Biases may be carried into the role, and often lack of clarity needed for maximum functioning exists. With the large caseloads of school counselors and the constant pull between direct and indirect service needs, the counselor's job may be one ideally suited for the role of consultant. The role of consultant necessitates task change and expansion.

In actual service delivery, the struggle to define one's role as consultant tends to create tension between the consultant and others who have expectations which differ and change. The role of consultant needs to be defined as the primary role. School psychologists have often led the way in the move to redefine their role (Fairchild, 1982; Alpert and Trachtman 1980; Lambert, Sandoval, and Corder, 1975). The activities include observation, assessment of classroom planning and program evaluation, translating pupil information to teachers, initiation of contact with a teacher, strategy intervention, curriculum development, and consultation sessions with parents.

The issue of role definition does not have easy answers. It is complicated by the expectation that the school psychologist and school counselor serve several publics. They must respond to the expectations of administrators, community, parents, teachers, and students. Often these publics have divergent expectations. Consequently, priorities must be determined for programs and services. Systematic efforts need to be used to implement these priorities. As roles are created, functions must be defined. Visible, well-defined, and carefully evaluated programs are needed in schools. Whether a school psychologist or a school counselor, the consultant needs to help others understand and appreciate the dimensions of this role. When consultation indeed comes first, other tasks necessary to accomplish will be administered in light of the consultation role.

The internal consultant has more potential for role conflict than the consultant coming from the outside. The outside consultant has contracted with the school for a specific task and, when that task is accomplished, the consultant will leave. No other roles will likely become entangled with the designated reason for the consultant's presence. This is especially true if the consultant has been careful to develop a clear, workable contract. This is less true for the inside consultant who will move from task to task attempting to meet a variety of expectations. Few of these expectations will be clearly laid out. Role conflict becomes a greater problem for the inside consultant. It is, in fact, a problem which has been addressed in some schools with the help of an outside consultant. The more conscious the inside consultant is of the potential confusion, the more the consultant is likely to work to develop clarity.

Relationship Issues

School consultants need to be aware of the relationship between themselves and their consultees. When the consultant is external to the system, he or she lacks familiarity of the territory; of the people; and of the institution, all of which impact on how the consultant is received and on the recommendations the consultant will eventually make. The consultant's main experience in schools may, in fact, be those from childhood. This places the consultant in a position of disadvantage and limits the use of a variety of skills. The consultant's limited view of the institution narrows perceptions. The consultant needs to become reacquainted with the school as an institution, using his/her objectivity, to become familiarized with the system.

Consultees, on the other side of the relationship, may be resistant to an outsider. A consultant from outside the system may be seen as someone who does not understand the system. Resistance may occur and barriers may be built due to a sense of threat, which makes collaboration difficult. When a teacher seeks help, the cost is often a sense of failure, as the experience may require acknowledgement of inadequacies. There is a sense of being alone in the classroom which may limit the exposure a teacher wants to feel. Vulnerability is difficult without a level of trust with the consultant. Teachers often feel they should be equally effective with every problem and with every student. When the orientation of the consultant is different from that of the teacher, tension between the two and especially in the teacher may permeate the relationship. If the consultant comes from within the school, the teacher needs to be told exactly what is the role of the consultant. This will necessitate a definition of confidentiality. When the consultant is outside, it is possible the consultant will make different usages of terms, approaches, biases, and academic orientation. For example, if a consultant uses psychological jargon unfamiliar to the teacher, the teacher could feel intimidated. The consultant needs to recognize the orientation of the consultee, which includes using terms that have meaning for the consultee.

The consultant needs to be familiarized with the system. Whether inside or outside, the consultant would do well to spend time assessing internal forces: the structure, the norms, communication, boundaries, and problem-solving mechanisms. Influential people, such as the principal, veteran, respected teachers, and secretaries, need to be identified. The consultant should acknowledge the network of people and committees when planning strategies (Gallessich, 1981). School norms must be considered. The consultant can discover, for example, whether or not teachers discuss classroom issues over lunch. One would not want to initiate such a discussion at such a time unless it is the usual habit of the school. Or, a consultant would want to learn if communications in the school are normally handled face-to-face or by written memo. These are all part of the acclimation process for the consultant. An analysis of the system is necessary in order to know how to be a part of the system.

Multicultural Influences

School consultants need to be sensitive to the influences of environmental, personal, and social–organizational factors upon the institution. Such variation exists among schools and within any school itself, and some differences necessitate departures from techniques the consultant has found effective. It may be necessary for the consultant to use flexibility and adaptability.

An understanding of the particular community and an ability to communicate with that community are essential characteristics for the consultant. Consultation programs and services are affected by the communication process. This process incorporates skills of listening with dimensions that are verbal, nonverbal, cognitive, and affective. The consultant needs to be diligent about these dimensions. Consultants should not be fooled by what appears to be a simplistic process. This is especially true in regards to multiculturalism. The communication- and relationship-building skills of the consultant will largely determine the success of the consultation. The consultant needs a critical awareness of the social and cultural nature of these relationship-building skills.

The school consultant's focus must be multicultural. Schools are often representative of our multicultural society. Yet frequently, the consultant represents one culture and the school another. Cultural awareness is very important for the consultant. This awareness needs to include, but not be limited to, racial and ethnic groups. It should include knowledge of cultural norms and stereotypes of other groups within society who have experienced discrimination. Implications of racism, sexism, classism, ageism, and handicapism all need to be studied.

The consultant has the responsibility to be aware of his/her personal culture—the values, concepts, beliefs, and principles of interaction—and how it may differ from that of the school or individual consultee(s). The consultant can then respond within the framework of two different perspectives, the consultant's and the school's. The consultant can demonstrate competencies within both cultures.

The recognition of multicultural issues in consultation programs is beneficial. Consultees can be taught to understand their own issues and biases and deal with these while working with clients. A model of effective consultation was developed (McIntosh and Coleman, 1984) wherein the target population was rural minority students. The purpose was to impact the decisions made regarding students by the school personnel. The model involved all adults in the school regardless of rank and responsibility. All staff participated in a total school effort using in-service programs. The training emphasized the elimination of nonfactual information and the provision of clear goals. The basic principle was to assist those persons involved in decision making regarding the student population. The staff was to divorce themselves, as much as possible, from their own biases, prejudices, value systems, and feelings when they were judging the behaviors of these particular students. The program was not designed to alter cultural values of the staff but to reduce the impact of those values when making decisions regarding the students.

There are many areas in which the consultant's attention to personal background, experience, and bias is important. One of the more critical and consuming is that of multiculturalism. Preparation for entering a system as consultant needs to include an understanding of the multicultural aspects of that system. This will impact heavily on the relationship and, consequently, the outcome of the consultation.

Resistance

The consultation process begins when the consultee requests assistance. In the case of schools, a teacher may approach a counselor to discuss a classroom problem. It is possible that instead of assistance, the teacher may want verification that a particularly difficult case cannot be resolved. It becomes a game (Curran, 1983) wherein coping with the problem has become too difficult for the teacher. The teacher may feel defeated by the student's behavior, so the teacher will make the case seem impossible to the consultant. The consultee lists all the difficulties and the numerous attempts made to resolve the problem case, often adding descriptions of the student's poor attitude. If the consultant joins in this defeatism, the game ensues, and what could be productive time is spent reinforcing the impossibility of the situation. The consultant is now in collusion with the consultee. The payoffs for the consultee are release from responsibility for the outcome of the case and sympathy from another professional.

The consultant's part of the game is important to note. It may be that the consultant has difficulty handling the teacher and, in addition, may feel incompetent to handle the difficult student. Consequently, the consultant joins the consultee in the game of misery over this case. By joining in the game, the consultant reinforces the teacher's thinking: the student is to blame for the poor outcome. The consultant is seen as supportive and helpful by not confronting the teacher on the game. The payoffs for the consultant are clear. The consultant need put little effort into the case since the student is "at fault," and the consultant is also rather popular with the teacher for his/her easy-going approach and the smooth relationships this creates. Both parties have an inflated sense of relief about the consultation sessions, convinced they did all they could in working toward resolution. Unfortunately, the student continues to experience the same set of difficulties—with a note in one's file stating two professionals agree that the problem is the student's, due to lack of initiation and/or motivation. Thus, the game is not only ineffective but misleading and likely to hurt. This type of game often occurs when the consultant is internal to the system. The consultant must face colleagues regularly and wish for smooth relationships to exist. However, the same pitfall exists for outside consultants as well. The outside consultant may take the easy route knowing she/he will not face the staff again and the consequences will not be hers or his.

The consultant can develop the consultation relationship in ways that avoid these pitfalls. An effective consultation process is enhanced by being aware of the interactional nature of the potential game. Since consultant and consultee contribute to the game, either can interrupt it. This interruption can best be done by refocusing on the client's problem and by keeping productivity the goal. The goal can be concretized by outlining specific problems and recommended interventions. If these are kept to descriptions of behaviors, the inclination to complain about the impossibility of the situation is minimized. The two participants need the security of a trusting relationship. Without trust, it becomes difficult for either consultant or consultee to work effectively. This will also contribute to a monitoring of the progress. The teacher is more likely to see this in a positive frame than unfavorably. Periodic checking provides for feedback between the two parties regarding satisfactions or dissatisfactions over details of the case. It also allows for a continued supportive relationship. Consultation may productively proceed in other areas.

Resistance occurs when the consultee avoids the problem-solving process with the consultant. Since change is considered a desirable outcome for consultation, it becomes important to assess the resistance to this change. At the administrative level, personnel may view consultative services with hesitancy, sensing changes may be called for in the status quo. Some personnel prefer the low risk of status quo over the unknown of change. With teachers, resistance may occur when they learn substantial involvement is necessary for effective consultation. They may be at the point of reducing their involvement rather than increasing responsibility. Inherent in the process of consultation is the tendency for the consultee to experience anxiety and, consequently, some level of resistance. Piersel and Gutkin (1983) have analyzed resistance to consultation in terms of rewards and punishments operative in the system. They suggest the issues connected to resistance result from the poor practice of consultation, not the models selected for the consultation. The practice or process is defined by the relationship between consultant and consultee. It is within a well-defined relationship that resistance can best be addressed and the issues resolved so that the consultation contract can be carried out. Relationship becomes key to many levels of consultation, including that of resistance.

CONTRACTING A CONSULTING RELATIONSHIP

The consultant–consultee relationship will be effectively developed within the structure of a contract. The contract, jointly developed, describes the goals for consultation; defines the problem(s); and includes the intervention strategies to be used. The consultant needs to be sure other aspects of the contract are clear. Inclusion of a time frame for consultation services and, if applicable, the reimbursements to the consultant are important. A description of the planned activities is appropriate for the contract as well as a mechanism for renegotiation and evaluation. A well-developed contract can provide the basis for evaluation.

In addition to the formal contract, the consultant and consultee need an agreement as to the process of the consultation sessions. The responsibility for managing the direction of the consultation sessions rests with the consultant. When the consultation is process oriented, the consultant and consultee work collaboratively. The consultant relies on the consultee for the details of the organizational structure, climate, and norms. The consultant is involved in mutual problem identification and resolution. The role of the consultant varies with the approach to consultation, and it is the responsibility of the consultant to remain within that role.

In contracting with a consultee the consultant needs to keep the discussion task-oriented and focused. For example, when the consultation is a client-centered approach, the emphasis needs to be kept on the client. Techniques such as asking the consultee to explore the history and background of the client, or to note the context of the occurrence of certain behaviors, assist in keeping to the contract. The message is communicated that the emphasis is on the client, rather than the consultee, and on the task-oriented process.

Consultation efforts may be misunderstood as counseling. The contract is for consultation. Yet, the two areas border at times and may cause uneasiness, especially in the consultee. A consultee may worry that problems with a client or the system may reflect on his/her own capabilities and that discussion of such personal matters would be painful, embarrassing, or uncomfortable. On the other hand, others welcome the opportunity to discuss and explore difficulties in every aspect of their lives. This may occur even after the consultant has clearly defined the limits of consultation. In this event, the consultant may confront the confines of the agreed-upon contract. The consultant needs to keep to the contract providing consultation and avoid offering psychotherapy. If counseling is needed, the consultant may refer the consultee for that purpose. Useful techniques for keeping to the consultation contract include asking mainly objective, nonpersonal questions; discussing problems by focusing on the client, not the consultee; controlling the consultee's anxiety about the case; and learning tactful interruptions when a consultee is disclosing too much personal information. Through repeated and consistent clarifications these topics fade away and it becomes clear to the consultee that the consultation session is not therapy. The consultee eventually learns that it is possible for consultation to cover a wide range of topics without undue invasion of privacy.

The consultation process requires clarity of role. It necessitates clarity not only of the role of the consultant, but also of the consultee. Thus, the process needs clarity and definition of purpose throughout. Goals of consultation need to exist. They do not need to be elaborate, but they must be clear and agreed upon by both parties. Use of a contract can help in the definition of role, purpose, and goals. It is most effective when the contract is written; this provides an easy way of reviewing the plan of action. The contract is a wise approach to an honest relationship between the consultant and consultee.

ETHICAL CONSIDERATIONS

School consultants do not have a particular set of rules that govern their behavior apart from those of their professional affiliation. For example, most school counselors belong to the American Association for Counseling and Development and would follow those ethical guidelines. No one set of guidelines exists, however, for all school consultants. This is true for both outside consultants and those inside the system. With all ethical concerns, it is wise for the consultant to give careful consideration to predictable problems before they arise. This allows the consultant some clarity of thought prior to taking action. The consultant needs some knowledge of ethical and legal responsibilities. These vary with the client population, the institution, and within the state in which the consultant is working. Ethically, the consultant is responsible to the hiring party, consultee, and client (Conoley and Conoley, 1982).

One of the primary ways a school consultant can exercise ethical behavior within the role is to promote professional attitudes and behaviors among the staff about confidentiality and informed consent. This includes being careful about the quality of the information found in written records as well as discussing problems of children and their families. The best approach is to focus on the strengths of clients and share information only with those who need to know in order to better educate the child. Ethical concerns are best expressed when everything said, or done, is with the best interest of the client in mind.

MODELS OF SCHOOL CONSULTATION

The consultation process may incorporate different models. Diagnostic interpretations are used in developing assumptions about the purpose of the consultation. The purpose and method of intervention lead to the selection of an appropriate model. It is important for the consultant to recognize varying needs of the consultee, which may necessitate the consultant using more than one model. The consultant can let the presenting problem guide the direction of the consultation and especially the choice of the model.

Three commonly used models in the school setting are: the mental health model, the medical model, and the behavior model. The mental health model is based on Gerald Caplan's (1970) four types of mental health consultation. The medical model is more traditional and may reflect the clinical orientation of many in the helping professions. The behavioral approach uses intervention strategies based on behavioral psychology. These and other models are described in Chapter 1.

Teacher preference for consultation models has been initially assessed by Curtis and Zins (1981). These authors express concern that little has been done to identify factors which might contribute to the consultee's use of the consultation service. Consultees are important in determining the success or failure of the consultative experience. Using the three models—medical/clinical, behavioral, and mental health—which specifically focus on consultee-centered case consultation, Curtis and Zins examined consultee preferences among 114 elementary school teachers. A Consultation Preference Instrument was designed to assess teacher preference for the three models. The teachers were asked to indicate preferences most attractive to them. Teacher preference results indicated 45.6 percent of the teachers preferred the behavior approach, 35.1 percent preferred the medical/clinical model, and 19.3 percent of the teachers preferred the mental health model. Curtis and Zins suggest there is a combined preference for the two models which comes from the mental health field: the behavioral and the mental health models. In both these models the consultant is not the expert. In both the teachers are encouraged toward more active participation by involving them in problem solving and planning. This result may show a move away from the more traditional model, which emphasizes the expertise of the consultant, toward collaborative models. However, it is important to identify possible reasons for the 35.1 percent of teachers who chose the medical/clinical model. That this model is the most traditional and the approach best known to teachers may be the major reason for such a large preference. Other reasons for this choice may be the teachers' desire to turn responsibility over to an expert or the desire for a rapid diagnosis and resolution which this model offers. Consultee perceptions of consultants are a more subtle indicator for their preferences. It is possible consultees select the model based on how they view the consultant administering the model. In any case, the wide distribution of choice for consultant models supports the notion that a consultant needs to be trained in more than one model.

Babcock and Pryzwansky (1983) reported consultation model preferences from elementary school principals, special education teachers, and elementary teachers. They looked at four models across five stages of the consultation process. The models were: collaborative, mental health, medical and expert. All three education groups rated the collaboration model above the others. The preference was consistent for the most part across the stages of consultation. The collaboration model relies on the relationship established between the consultant and consultee. Developing and maintaining a working relationship takes time. Once this occurs, further consultant–consultee experiences are facilitated. However, it may be viewed as an initial disadvantage due to the time invested in the early stages.

Jason and Ferone (1978) compared the process model to the behavioral model and found the behavioral approach to be the most effective in reducing problem behaviors during the intervention and follow-up period. Techniques used in the behavioral model may be especially effective at the time of intervention. The techniques are designed to effect and maintain behavior changes. The behavioral model seems especially well designed to deal with client-centered cases.

Fedner, Biacchi, and Duffey (1979) studied consultative strategies ranked by special education teachers. They found that special education teachers' favored strategies related to assisting the child over and above the strategies for teacher assistance. These preferred child-oriented strategies involved explaining techniques to alleviate the child's difficulties and describing dynamics of the child's problem. The consultant spent time discussing new techniques which could be used with the child. In addition, the consultant processed the dynamics of the child's problem, such as discussing family dynamics and the implications on the child. Special education teachers often have developed skills in behavior change; consequently, they need consultation in other areas. Intervention can be rather brief, using the medical model, or more time can be spent with the consultee, developing a holistic understanding of the child's dynamics using the process model.

A combination of the process model which incorporates a collaborative approach and the behavioral model emphasizing intervention techniques may prove to be useful in many school situations. The process model allows the consultant to develop a comprehensive approach to the identified problem and any associated concerns. It provides a place for the incorporation of consultee needs. The behavioral approach is useful in addressing the problem initially defined. This model is designed to focus on the specific concern the teacher has for the child. Thus combining these two models can give the school consultant flexibility needed in addressing a wide range of concerns in the school.

Client-centered consultation featuring behavior modification techniques and consultee-centered consultation were used together to help modify the behavior of disruptive students in school (Meyers, 1975). The teacher's feelings about being the authority figure in the classroom were addressed in consultee-centered consultation that increased the effectiveness of teaching. This intervention was followed by measurable changes in the behavior of children in the classroom. The combination of addressing client problems using the behavioral model and identifying consultation concerns of the teacher, offers a comprehensive approach for the school consultant. The time spent with the consultee will not only assist in resolving immediate concerns but enables the consultee to develop new skills which enhance the management or prevention of future problems. Any skill development in an initial consultation experience offers the teacher tools which can be used later. These tools may very well reduce referrals by the teacher as the teacher better handles the problems in the classroom.

The work of Conoley and Conoley (1982) studied the effectiveness of a client-centered consultative approach on the quality of the consultees' problem description and remedial plan development. Skills in describing classroom problems and generating appropriate remedial plans were measured. They found consultation with and without consultant observation were effective in improving problem identification skills. The consultation with observation, however, achieved better problem descriptions in a shorter period of time than the group without consultant observation. Observation by the consultant is a tool used by school consultants in a variety of models. Initially, it may increase the consultant's time with the teacher; however, it appears to have long-term benefits. Future considerations and goals may be facilitated with a skillful teacher's problem identification abilities.

An additional method focused on consultees involves skill development. In-service training programs for school staff, especially teachers, may improve the use of consultation. Knoff (1985) reports an in-service and consultation program for educational staffs which has four interacting units: value clarification, models of discipline, techniques and related issues, and problem-solving practice. Other training experiences may be more informal, such as problem identification. Teachers may have the opportunity to describe cases and receive assistance from the consultant in identifying problems. Rogeness, Stokes, Bednar, and Gorman (1977) found training teachers in defining specific adequate and inadequate behaviors can be a useful tool in entry. Clear definition of behaviors assists the consultant in understanding the problem and accelerates the process on to intervention. In-service teacher training is an appropriate consultation approach and can upgrade the consultees in a variety of teacher functions.

The consultant needs to know a wide range of models and evaluate the use of these models. The chosen models can be influenced by consultee preference and the presenting problem. Consultants are best prepared to offer needed services to a wider group of consultees with divergent needs if they are trained in more than one model. In this way, the consultant is able to adapt to consultee preference and respond to various presenting problems. Exclusive use of one approach for all situations may prove ineffective. Exploration of the impact of various interactions on populations such as the culturally diverse student is an important direction for consultants.

The consultant can use the understanding and application of human behavior theories to assess cognitive and affective dimensions of the client, consultee, and system. The development of the relationship is an integral part of the process and should enhance the use of any model. Consultants who understand the system, the client population, the consultee population, and who have an understanding of a variety of applicable models and know their own beliefs and attitudes, are able to begin a productive consultation process.

DIRECTIONS FOR RESEARCH

Research is needed in the areas of multicultural implications for consultation. Multicultural implications have a great deal to do with biases, values, and attitudes. They also impact on the consultant–consultee relationship.

The collaborative working relationship is dependent on the relating ability of these partners. Consequently, research is necessary to consider the pairing of the various characteristics and qualities found in multicultural studies.

It may be that we need to turn our attention more clearly to the role of the school consultant. A move away from the emphasis on models is timely, yet we want to retain what we have learned about school consultation models. We have a considerable amount of quite helpful material on models (Fairchild, 1982; Alpert, Ballantyne, and Griffiths, 1981; and Alpert and Trachtman, 1980; Knoff, 1985; and Jason and Ferone, 1978). We need to use this data and develop a clearer concept of the role of a consultant in the school. In addition, we can focus on the consultation relationship and study the dynamics between the consultant and the consultee. Meyers, Freidman, Gaughan, and Pitt (1978) suggest the need for intensive study of small numbers of consultation relationships, replicated reliably many times, so that researchers can generalize their conclusions. The authors' concern is in the lack of research to identify what happens at the affective level of consultation. There have not been enough attempts to identify relevant feelings and attitudes or to consider the relationship of these affective variables to the consultation outcome.

Other approaches to the research of consultation include the maintenance of behavior change (Barbrack, 1980). Behavior change has been studied; however, the factors contributing to the maintenance of change have not been evaluated clearly enough. Also, more studies relating process variables to outcome are indicated, as are programmatic studies and studies incorporating more experimental controls and the utilization of follow-up data (Alpert and Yammer, 1983).

There is a need to collect data on more than one party in the consultation process. Typically, data is obtained on the client when the process is client-centered, or on the consultee when consultee-centered. Alpert and Yammer (1983) suggest data needs to be collected on client, consultee, consultant, and system variables. If this approach was used, it is conceivable that the aspects mentioned above could be integrated. Studies could be comprehensive and include the assessment of consultee–consultant relationships and the impact of multiculturalism.

SUMMARY

The school consultant's role, influenced by PL 94–142 and expectations from administration, faculty, and parents, is marked with change. The consultant is called to broaden what has been a traditional role of direct service to incorporate indirect service to a variety of populations. Teacher consultation allows the consultant to be a resource person for the teacher and assist him/her in developing skills that enhance classroom environment and learning. Parent consultation may be used in conjunction with teacher consultation or as a program alone. It is helpful in reducing parent confusion and resistance and increasing parent awareness and assistance. The consultant's role is appropriate to working with a team of school personnel or with the administration regarding school concerns. The school consultant's role is marked by role conflict and confusion which can best be resolved by identifying priorities for programs and services.

REFERENCES

ALPERT, J., BALLANTYNE, D., and GRIFFITHS, D. (1981). Characteristics of consultants and consultees and success in mental health consultation. *Journal of School Psychology*, 19 (4), 312–322.

ALPERT, J., and TRACHTMAN, G. (1980). School psychological consultation in the eighties: Relevance for the delivery of special services. *School Psychological Review*, 9 (3), 234–238.

ALPERT, J., and YAMMER, M. (1983). Research in school consultation: A content analysis of selected journals. *Professional Psychology: Research and Practice*, 14 (5), 604–612.

BABCOCK, N., and PRYZWANSKY. (1983). Models of consultation: Preferences of educational professionals at five stages of service. *Journal of School Psychology*, 21 (3), 359–366.

BARBRACK, C. (1980). Program consultation: A framework for development and improvement of special education and related services. *School Psychology Review*, 9 (3), 239–2246.

BERGAN, J., and TOMBARI, M. (1976). Consultant skill and efficiency and the implementation and outcomes of consultation. *Journal of School Psychology*, 2, 3–13.

BERGER, N. (1979). Beyond testing: A decision-making system for providing school psychological consultation. *Professional Psychology*, June, 273–277.

BONEBRAKE, C., and BORGERS, S. (1984). Counselor role as perceived by counselors and principals. *Elementary School Guidance and Counseling*, February, 194–199.

CAPLAN, G. (1970). *The theory and practice of mental health consultation*. New York: Basic Books.

CONOLEY, J., and CONOLEY, C. (1982). The effects of two conditions of client-centered consultation on student teacher problem descriptions and remedial plans. *Journal of School Psychology*, 20 (4), 323–328.

CURRAN, J. (1983). Potential pitfalls of a teacher–counselor consultation game. *Elementary School Guidance and Counseling*, February, 231–233.

CURTIS, M., and WATSON, K. (1980). Changes in consultee problem clarification skills following consultation. *Journal of School Psychology*, 18 (3), 210–221.

CURTIS, M., and ZINS, J. (1981). *The theory and practice of school consultation*. Springfield, IL: Charles C. Thomas.

DICKINSON, D., and ADCOX, S. (1984). Program evaluation of a school consultation program. *Psychology in the Schools*, 21, July, 336–342.

DINKMEYER, D. JR., and DINKMEYER, D. SR. (1984). School counselors as consultants in primary prevention programs. *The Personnel and Guidance Journal,* April, 464–466.

FAIRCHILD, T. (1982). The school psychologist's role as an assessment consultant. *Psychology in the Schools,* 19, 200–208.

FEDNER, M., BIACCHI, A., and DUFFEY, J. (1979). Priorities of special education teachers regarding consultative strategies. *Psychological Reports,* 44, 1181–1182.

FISHER, L. (1986). Systems-based consultation with schools. In L. Wynne, S. McDaniel, and T. Weber, (eds.), *Systems consultation: A new perspective for family therapy* (342–356). New York: The Guilford Press.

GALLESSICH, J. (1981). Organizational factors influencing consultation in schools. In M. Curtis, and J. Zins, (eds.), *The theory and practice of school consultation.* Springfield, IL: Charles C. Thomas.

GUTKIN, T., and AJCHENBAUM, M. (1984). Teacher's perceptions of control and preferences for consultative services. *Professional Psychology: Research and Practice,* 15 (4), 565–570.

HAIGHT, S., and MOLITOR, D. (1983). A survey of special education teacher consultants. *Exceptional Children,* 49 (6), 23–25.

HANSEN, J. (1977). Prevention through teacher consultation. *The Journal of School Health,* May, 289–292.

JASON, L., and FERONE, L. (1978). Behavioral versus process consultation interventions in school settings. *American Journal of Community Psychology,* 6 (6), 531–543.

KNOFF, H. (1985). Discipline in the schools: An inservice and consultation program for educational staffs. *The School Counselor,* January, 211–218.

KRATOCHWILL, T. (1985). Selection of target behaviors in behavioral consultation. *Behavioral Assessment,* 7, 49–61.

LAMBERT, M., SANDOVAL, J., and CORDER, R. (1975). Teacher perceptions of school-based consultants. *Professional Psychology,* May, 204–216.

McINTOSH, D., and COLEMAN, Y. (1984). Effective consultation about minority students in rural communities. *Elementary School Guidance and Counseling,* 18 (4), 303–307.

MEDWAY, F. (1979). How effective is school consultation?: A review of recent research. *The Journal of School Psychology,* 17, 275–282.

MEYERS, J. (1975). Consultee-centered consultation with a teacher as a technique in behavior management. *American Journal of Community Psychology,* 3 (2), 111–121.

MEYERS, J., FREIDMAN, M., GAUGHAN, E., and PITT, N. (1978). An approach to investigate anxiety and hostility in consultee-centered consultation. *Psychology in the Schools,* April, 15 (2), 292–296.

PIERSEL, W., and GUTKIN, T. (1983). Resistance to school-based consultation: A behavioral analysis of the problem. *Psychology in the Schools,* 20, July, 311–320.

RITTER, D. (1978). Effects of a school consultation program upon referral patterns of teachers. *Psychology in the Schools,* 15, 239–242.

ROGENESS, G., STOKES, J., BEDNAR, R., and GORMAN, B. (1977). School intervention program to increase behaviors and attitudes that promote learning. *Journal of Community Psychology,* 5, 246–256.

STEWART-LESTER, K. (1982). Increased consultation opportunities for school psychologists: A service delivery model. *Psychology in the Schools,* 19, 86–91.

CHAPTER FOUR
CONSULTING IN BUSINESS AND INDUSTRY

During the past decade an increasing number of mental health professionals have become interested in consulting in business and industry. Business and industry would seem to possess problems relevant to the mental health consultant's expertise as well as the financial resources to pay for that expertise. The latter concern is particularly noteworthy as governmental funding of mental health services has stabilized or decreased. Mental health professionals have found opportunities in business and industry and become involved in a range of programs, including Employee Assistance Programs (EAPs; Toomer, 1982) and psychotherapy for executives (Much, 1984).

This chapter will address the key issues around mental health consulting in business and industry. Surveys of mental health consultants' experiences in business and industry will be reported along with data concerning the use of such consultants. Next, examples of mental health consulting in these fields will be presented. Important issues that are likely to face the mental health consultant in these settings are discussed. Finally, strategies for preparing for mental health consulting in business and industry are presented.

INTEREST IN MENTAL HEALTH CONSULTATION

In general, mental health consultants' interest in business settings appear to exceed business people's interest in hiring such consultants. For example, Toomer (1982) assessed the level of interest of psychologists in business and industry by means of a survey sent to 1,000 members of the American Psychological Association. Three hundred and seventy persons returned usable responses; Toomer was interested in the responses of the 104 persons in this group who were counseling psychologists. Only 3 percent were employed in manufacturing or business settings, but 73 percent reported moderate to high interest in expanding their work in business. In fact, 38 percent reported being very interested in business, exceeding the group's reported interest for working in health care, mental health agencies, public schools, research, and education. This high degree of interest in business consulting is likely to be generalizable across the mental health professions.

Barkway and Kirby (1983) surveyed personnel managers to learn about their use of and attitudes toward mental health consultants. They sent questionnaires to a random sample of 325 managers in companies (primarily manufacturing) employing 200 or more people; 130 usable responses were received, a return rate of 40 percent. Half of the respondents reported having the authority to hire an industrial psychologist; those having this authority were also more likely to have a college degree.

Comparing their survey to one conducted 10 years earlier, Barkway and Kirby (1983) reported a slight increase in the number of companies using psychological testing (from 38 percent to 46 percent). Testing areas included (in order of most frequent use) special aptitudes, personality, intelligence, vocational, and interpersonal skills. Respondents indicated that such tests were employed for personnel selection, promotion, counseling, and clinical assessment. However, they found no increase over the past decade in the number of companies (around 20 percent) actually employing an industrial psychologist. Only 10 percent of the companies hired a psychologist full-time, while 14 percent hired a part-time psychologist. The vast majority (76 percent) hired a consultant.

Barkway and Kirby also provided data regarding the managers' attitudes toward industrial psychologists. Managers expressed mixed opinions: while about half felt psychologists could contribute to productivity and job satisfaction, only one-third considered it desirable to have an industrial psychologist in their company. Managers considered such areas as recruitment, screening, test administration, personnel evaluation, motivation studies, communication effectiveness, and job satisfaction assessment to be beneficial services that could be provided by consultants.

Managers still do not perceive a strong need for mental health consultants in their company, Barkway and Kirby conclude. As a result, consultants must sell management on the usefulness of their skills. They suggest that consultants use business publications to increase managers' awareness of mental health consultation as well as to learn more about business settings.

ROLES AND EXAMPLES

All consultants are assumed to offer organizations objectivity, methods for overcoming resistance to change, analytic skill, time, and sensitivity to organizational issues (Wells, 1983). In addition, mental health consultants offer specialized knowledge for understanding individuals, interpersonal relationships, and organizational systems. Consultants typically proceed through the process by following a general model. This often includes strategies for gaining entry into the organization, problem identification, goal setting, choice and implementation of strategies, and evaluation and termination (Brown, 1985).

Toomer (1982) provides an overview of the various settings in which mental health consultants may play a role. These include: (1) personnel departments, where consultants may provide help with career counseling, termination, suitability for transfer, employee attitudes, and assessment of work-related stress; (2) medical care, including the diagnosis of work-related medical problems with psychosomatic components; (3) equal employment opportunity, including the development or evaluation of fair assessment devices; (4) safety, including the effects of stress and alcohol on accident rates; (5) labor relations, including negotiations, teaching of listening skills, confrontation, assertiveness, and conflict resolution; (6) training, including updating of employee skills; and (7) Employee Assistance Programs (EAPs), including chemical dependency programs, family problems, job performance, and absenteeism. Regarding item 7, organizing and working in EAPs have tended to be highly publicized roles for mental health consultants. Consultants in EAPs typically offer short-term treatment for the problems mentioned above or make referrals to other mental health practitioners and agencies in the community.

Osipow (1982) describes consulting roles similar to those presented by Toomer: (1) career development, including retirement preparation and changing unproductive work behavior; (2) selection of personnel; and (3) clinical issues, including the stress of split work roles, job loss, and family counseling. Osipow also notes that consultants could be useful in helping the white-collar professional deal with Type A behavior as well as the blue-collar worker cope with repetitive work. Type A behavior refers to a type of psychological stress in which the individual typically experiences considerable time pressure (often self-imposed) as well as hostility toward others. Treatment of persons exhibiting Type A behavior often involves changing attitudes about the importance of work, teaching relaxation skills, and group counseling (e.g., Roskies, Seraganian, Oseasohn, Smilga, Martin, and Hanley, 1989). Repetitive work occurs in settings like factories where employees must complete simple tasks at a fast pace; intervention might include teaching relaxation skills or job restructuring (e.g., better spacing of work breaks, increased teamwork, or job switching).

Oskamp's (1988) list of nontraditional employment opportunities for applied psychologists is generalizable to other mental health professionals. He notes that consultants may be employed in: (1) consumer and media research and marketing; (2) computer consulting, planning, and management; (3) energy and resource conservation research; (4) environmental design and habitability; and (5) the traditional consulting positions in organizational behavior research and development. Oskamp notes that for positions as organizational consultants, mental health professionals "may need to broaden their skills and market them aggressively in order to compete successfully with graduates of professional schools of management or business" (p. 484). He suggests field work or an internship in a relevant setting as a prerequisite for full-time employment or consulting.

In additional to content areas such as career counseling and training of interviewing skills, mental health consultants vary in their philosophy about what types of interventions are appropriate for consultation activities. The simplest method of consulting is to transfer the skills of individual counseling and psychotherapy from the clinic to the corporation. For example, Much (1984) reports a consulting arrangement in which executives are persuaded "to perceive their business as a unit of interrelationships that closely mirrors relationships they have or have had with their own families" (p. 88). In other words, Much's consultants have the task of translating the material of individual therapy—for example, recognizing the influence of family patterns on one's interpersonal relationships—into corporate consulting. For example, a manager in an advertising agency, whose father was very domineering and rigid, might constrain the creativity and productivity of her employees by adopting and enforcing a set of regulations regarding dress, clocking in and out of work, and work breaks. The consultant's job, then, would be to function as a therapist, helping the manager explore her past relationships and connect those insights to her current work behavior. In such a manner the manager might become more flexible and thereby increase her employees' effectiveness.

Many consultants, however, view personal counseling as inappropriate. In fact, they interpret requests for personal counseling by consultees as being indicative of resistance (Randolph, 1985; Caplan, 1970). From this perspective, personal counseling is irrelevant to addressing organizational issues. Randolph (1985) suggests that expressions of negative affect by the consultee ("I'm really dissatisfied with this company") are subtle requests for personal counseling and should be deemphasized by the consultant in favor of attention to the identified consultation problem (e.g., increasing departmental teamwork).

Just as group counseling offers advantages for some clients in terms of efficiency and impact over one-to-one work (cf. Yalom, 1985), individual counseling in a corporate setting may be a less efficient and less powerful means of providing assistance. Staff and organizational development approaches treat companies as systems which require intervention. Improving these systems is likely to help individuals within the organization as well as increase the organization's efficiency as a whole.

Taking a systems approach, Czander (1986) suggests that problems can develop if consultants simply focus on one *department* within an organization. He notes that the consultant is often called to intervene with a deviant department or subsystem after other portions of the organization complain. Two problems can occur if the consultant then intervenes with just the offending department: (1) the department is likely to perceive the consultant as an enemy, and (2) the consultant fails to recognize the functional role of the deviant subsystem in maintaining the status quo of the organization. The systems consultant, Czander maintains, would want to know both why the organization cannot manage the department itself and "why . . . they [are] content in blaming rather than understanding that they (the conglomerate) may in fact be a contributor to this dysfunctional division" (p. 194).

Czander (1986) suggest that one of the methods the consultant may employ to become educated about the organization is to pay particular attention to the relationship between consultee and consultant. For example, if the consultant has difficulty gaining clarity about what the consultee wants from the consultation, this may be an indicator of ambivalence or resistance to outside help.

Argyris (1970; 1971; cited in Ziegenfuss and Lasky, 1980) sees organizational development as a process of obtaining valid information, helping the client to make a positive adjustment to organizational diagnosis, and getting the client to make a commitment to change. Dustin and Blocher (1984) describe organizational development as interventions designed to affect system functioning rather than individual functioning. They indicate that organizational development typically involves collection of data from an organization's members (e.g., through surveys and questionnaires) and then providing feedback to the organization about this information. Data collection is often part of organizational development, but it may not be employed to evaluate the outcome of the consultation. An assumption of this approach is that management may be unaware of problems (and creative solutions) known by employees at different levels of the organization (Greiner and Metzger, 1983). In fact, Greiner and Metzger state that "[t]he larger the organization, the less likely is bad news to reach the top" (p. 221).

For example, a consulting firm hired by a corporation to evaluate management practices may begin by administering a questionnaire designed to elicit employees' perceptions regarding the organization's goals, strengths and weaknesses, and relationships with managers. The consultant may review this information and then schedule small group sessions with employees to probe further about difficulties with a specific manager or to gather suggestions for improving communication. Finally, the consultant would compile and summarize this information (perhaps through tables of questionnaire results or selected comments) and present it to management for further consideration. McCormack and DeVore (1986) report on a similar process (described below under Improving the Work Climate) which was designed to collect data about a staff's perception of the chief of a Veteran's Administration psychology service.

Consultants as Managers

Other examples of consultants' roles in business and industry include the following. Demuth, Yates, and Coates (1984) indicate that mental health professionals, working as managers, may be able to improve the health and productivity of their employees. Consultants in managerial positions, they note, "need administrative know-how, political savvy, interpersonal effectiveness, personal effectiveness, personal 'presence,' leadership skills, perseverance, and a sense of mission" (p. 759). They suggest that industry provides new venues for applying psychological principles and advancing the science of psychology in evaluative research, health promotion, and primary prevention. Demuth and colleagues advise mental health professionals that "in an evolving professional world, it is either manage or be managed" (p. 767).

It is not at all uncommon, for example, to see mental health professionals in higher education move into positions as deans and administrators. These professionals continue to employ their knowledge about effective human interaction while learning about the administrative aspects of their new positions. If the career path of counselor to administrator has been successfully (and frequently) navigated in school settings, why should the mental health consultant not enjoy the same success as a manager in business and industry?

Employee-Assistance Programs

EAPs remain a primary source of opportunity for mental health consultants. EAPs began with concerns about alcohol, and these problems probably remain the largest source for referrals (Brill, Herzberg, and Speller, 1985). EAPs can also help troubled employees who have conflicts with supervisors, absenteeism, substance abuse, family discord, legal difficulties, and financial problems.

Brill and colleagues (1985) report that some estimates indicate that 20 to 30 percent of all absenteeism and 65 to 80 percent of all firings result from psychological difficulties. Studies have shown EAPs to increase attendance among troubled employees, decrease work compensation and health care costs, and reduce grievances and disciplinary actions. Toomer (1982) cites studies demonstrating the success of EAPs in increasing productivity and decreasing illness with alcoholics as well as the general benefits of mental health services versus costs. Toomer reports that EAPs have been shown to "reduce absenteeism, lower the number of sick claims, and improve safety performance and overall productivity" (p. 16).

Self-referral is the most common means of contacting an EAP, followed by supervisory referral of an impaired employee (Brill et al., 1985). Greiner and Metzger (1983) also describe a consultant, hired to design an alcoholism program, who found participants for the program by checking time-clock records to determine which employees were chronically late. If counseling is provided to troubled employees, it tends to be short-term, referring long-term cases to outside professionals. Confidentiality is particularly important in EAP settings. Most mental health consultants keep separate records on clients, and communication with supervisors is handled by having employees sign release-of-information statements (Brill et al., 1985).

Staff and Organizational Development

Aplin (1985) notes several trends which portend opportunities for mental health consultants in organizational development. The first trend, toward smaller organizations, refers to drastic reductions in the work forces of institutions. Consultants may help employees in these smaller groups deal with the increased personal stress and general pressure in the work environment. The second trend, toward egalitarian social and organizational values, suggests that consultants employ methods like team building to increase organizational effectiveness. Stern (1982) also observes this latter trend, suggesting that a number of influences have convinced most companies that "they must commit themselves to a more people-oriented work place" (p. 37). Mental health consultants, with their training in communication skills and group processes, would appear highly qualified to foster dialogues among employees and managers that replace hierarchical command structures.

Hipple and Ramsay (1985) reported on the use of quality circles to improve morale, absenteeism, and communication among 100 university dining service employees. They observe that quality circles "change the organizational atmosphere by offering food for thought and encouraging people to think and talk about the organization at other times" (p. 557). In Hipple and Ramsay's study, a consultant served as a group facilitator for biweekly meetings. Topics included the positive aspects of the work group, changes needed to make the group better, and how the group could work together better as a team. Employees' comments were later summarized and posted on a bulletin board. Hipple and Ramsay also suggest that consultants train employees on the use of consultation as a way of avoiding resistance and confusion.

Improving the Work Climate

A good example of a consultation designed to improve the work climate is provided by McCormack and DeVore (1986). They report on a program-centered consultation at a Veteran's Administration psychology service. The head of the unit felt that he was perceived as too coercive and asked the consultant to collect data from the psychology staff about the work climate. The consultants collected interview and survey data from each of the staff members. Anonymity was maintained for respondents and a written summary of findings was provided for all to review. The consultants viewed distribution of their report to *all* staff as crucial to the success of their consultation.

McCormack and DeVore found that staff perceived themselves as excluded from decision-making process. This was reflected in mistrust among levels of the organization. In response, the consultants scheduled monthly meetings between chief and staff. The consultants reported that they focused their efforts on creating a safe environment and acting as process observers who discussed how the group went about its business. The consultants were especially prepared to promptly interrupt and change destructive interpersonal transactions.

McCormack and DeVore evaluated the results of their evaluation using Moos's (1981) Work Environment Scales (WES). They suggest that such evaluations are better conducted with broad-band instruments "that assess many dimensions of social climate that are pertinent to satisfaction and productivity than [with] a more narrowly focused assessment approach" (p. 56). Pre- and posttesting (eight months following initial assessment) using the WES demonstrated improvement in work climate, including higher ratings of supervisory support, job autonomy, task orientation, and job clarity. A two-year follow-up indicated a significant increase in job satisfaction.

McCormack and DeVore's *evaluation* of their consultation efforts is unusual. Many consultants do not systematically assess the effectiveness of their work. While consultants often include some type of data gathering as part of problem definition, Czander (1986) suggests that the most serious deficiency in the field of consulting is the lack of evaluation of consultation interventions.

Stress Management

Mental health consultants are uniquely qualified to help individuals and organizations design strategies to decrease stress and burnout. Prolonged stress is presumed to affect how employees interact with co-workers, employers, and clients (see Jackson, 1984; Grol, Mokkink, Smits, Van Eijk, Beek, Mesker, and Mesker-Niesten, 1985) and to increase absenteeism, turnover, and health problems (Meier, 1983; Jackson, 1984). Jackson (1984) suggests a staff development approach which teaches: (1) new employees to have realistic (i.e., lowered) expectations about their work in order to avoid disillusionment, perhaps through an orientation program; (2) conflict resolution and negotiation; and (3) openness to job change on the part of both employee and employer. Organizational interventions which should decrease stress include increased employee participation in decision-making, increased feedback about job performance, reduced role conflict and ambiguity, support groups, and persuading managers to be more open to feedback from employees (Jackson, 1984).

Research

Levy-Leboyer (1988) describes the use of a French consulting team to research and provide recommendations regarding vandalism of public telephone booths. The telephone department staff believed that such destruction was primarily the result of thieves and juvenile delinquents. Consultants' interviews with delinquents, however, indicated that while this group approved of theft if motivated by such needs as hunger or social inequality, they disapproved of vandalism, "which they described as an aggressive and destructive act without any justification" (p. 782). Vandals, however, disapproved of any form of robbery, but "they approved of vandalism of public property both because it had a symbolic value and because it did not harm any specific person" (p. 782).

The consultants then proceeded to unobtrusively observe the most vandalized booths. They initially found that persons who vandalized the phones did so when the phones did not work or would not return money.

Customers then attempted to fix the telephone by shaking or hitting it; if these actions failed, some customers then became frustrated and damaged the phone. The consultants then began to systematically gather data at the booths, completing 518 observations where customers' characteristics and behavior in the booths were recorded. A survey of 200 telephone customers was also completed, with 55 percent indicating that they felt angry when faced with a broken telephone and 69 percent admitting to shaking the inoperative phone. The observational and survey research indicated that much of the vandalism was performed by ordinary citizens, not delinquents or thieves.

Levy-Leboyer notes that the telephone staff received this information with interest despite the fact that the results made the *staff*, not thieves and delinquents, at least partially responsible for the vandalism. The consultants, in collaboration with the staff, designed a poster to show customers where to find another street phone and how to get lost money back. This poster was then placed in a series of booths where the phones had been taken out of service for one day. Observations of this new system showed a marked decrease in vandalism.

Levy-Leboyer reports that the telephone department then discontinued the poster idea. While the consultants managed to convince the company's technical people of the need for the new information poster, they did not change the attitudes of higher management. Management remained convinced that deviant persons were committing the vandalism. Thus, the telephone company adopted a card system instead of coins, believing that removal of the money box would deter vandalism. However, Levy-Leboyer notes that "this new telephone is frequently vandalized—when it is out of order" (p. 783).

ISSUES

One of the most important issues that face mental health consultants who desire to work in business and industry is the clash of interests and values between the two professions. It is clear that considerable potential exists for power struggles between mental health consultant and business consultee.

At one end of the spectrum are the desires of some mental health consultants to humanize business and industry. For example, Ridley and Hellervik (1982) suggest that consultants should promote "productive individuals in humane organizational environments" (p. 54). Similarly, Demuth and colleagues (1984) believe that managing does not mean being "guided exclusively by profit motives" (p. 760). Ridley and Hellervik also indicate, however, that mental health consulting may not be viewed by business people as a legitimate activity, at least in terms of profit. The result, they suggest, is that mental health consultants will continue to play a small, restricted role in business and industry.

Whatever their motivation, mental health consultants must contribute in some way to the bottom line. For example, Toomer (1982) notes that some managers, particularly those who are more oriented toward business or hard science, may request confidential information about employees. Such managers must be educated, Toomer suggests, as to the information to which they have and don't have access. However, Toomer concludes that such managers are less likely to challenge consultants whose activities contribute to the company profits.

This conflict goes so far as to affect suggestions about the titles that mental health consultants employ. Discussing the potential role of counseling psychologists as business consultants, Ridley and Hellervik (1982) suggest that counseling psychologists substitute "consulting" for "counseling" in their title. They maintain that individuals who talk with a "consultant" are likely to be perceived by themselves and others as fully functioning, whereas individuals who converse with "counselors" are weak and sick. Ridley and Hellervik conclude that "it is unlikely that 'counselors' will ever have a significant function in an organization where power, achievement, and overall competence is highly valued by the potential clientele, and the projection of these qualities is central to achieving the major rewards dispensed by organizations" (p. 53). Presumably, this advice would hold for other mental health consultants as well (e.g., consulting psychiatrist, social worker).

Wilbur and Vermilyea (1982) believe that mental health consultants will always remain on the fringe of business and will not become part of the decision-making process. They suggest that mental health consultants see themselves less as counselors and more as business people. In business, they suggest, mental health services must be continuously sold and justified.

Wilbur and Vermilyea (1982) suggest that mental health consultants with a research background must be especially ready to adapt to the business setting. A conflict is likely between "the scientists's inclination to collect 'just a little more information' . . . [and] the businessperson's need to act now" (p. 32). They observe that business people typically act on the basis of far less evidence than scientists usually do. The implication of Wilbur and Vermilyea's discussion is that mental health consultants must be willing to suspend or discard a substantial portion of their professional identity, be that researcher or counselor.

On the other hand, Osipow (1982) suggests that business decision-makers need to change their attitudes toward counseling in industry. Some managers view psychology as a fuzzy field unconcerned with real problems; similarly, some workers try to avoid contact with the "company shrink." Osipow notes that business exists for profit and so tends to take a different view of employees than mental health professionals traditionally do. He suggests that consultants may be better served by presenting their ability to service the "human resources" of business and industry. Business is certainly concerned with the service of its technological and mechanical capacity, and such an analogy may help explain how mental health consultants could be useful.

Conflicts can also arise concerning the role of the consultant in decision making. Siver (1983) notes that in a highly specialized area, the consultant may best understand the problem and may be the best person to decide on a proper course of action. Siver advises managers, however, to avoid using consultants as decision makers. Siver believes that one of the wrong reasons for hiring a consultant is to make a decision. Instead, consultants should help problem-solve and recommend practical solutions.

Decision making can be a trap for both consultees and consultants. Consultees who find consultants' recommendations unpleasant may insure that the consultants have no role in decision making. On the other hand, consultees who do not wish to bear responsibility for implementing risky decisions may lure the consultant into decision-making responsibilities, only to later place blame for problems onto the consultant.

Hirsch (in Stern, 1982) suggests that 70 percent of consultants' potential clients have some resistance to mental health consultants but could be persuaded to use such services. Such individuals may be difficult to work with, however. On the other hand, Gavin (1977) advises that mental health consultants simply treat business's antipathy as resistance to be worked through.

PREPARATION AND EXPECTATIONS

A number of strategies have been recommended for graduate students and mental health professionals who wish to pursue consulting in business and industry. For example, Demuth and colleagues (1984) suggest the development of managerial expertise through informal support systems, mentors, continuing education (from such sources as the American Management Association), interdisciplinary management training (such as seeking a second degree like an MBA), and pre- and postdoctoral training in academic departments. Ridley and Hellervik (1982) also suggest that traditional graduate training be complemented with training in business administration or management.

Stark and Romans (1982) suggest that persons considering business consulting develop experience in such areas as: (1) managing or supervising others; (2) performing group-level or systems interventions; (3) designing courses and programs; (4) evaluating programs; (5) managing a budget; (6) terminating another's employment; (7) working with computers; (8) dealing with professionals in other disciplines; (9) developing a person's potential in terms of productivity; and (10) performing research in business and industry. As part of their graduate training, many students in counseling-related professions are likely to have training in areas 1 and 2. Students who work as teaching assistants or in outreach and prevention programs will gain experience in 3 and 9, while their efforts with master's theses and dissertations will provide an introduction to the areas described in 4, 7, and 10. Typical graduate programs in mental health will provide the least exposure to 5, managing a budget, 6, terminating another's employment, 8, dealing with professionals in other disciplines, and 9, developing a person's potential in terms of productivity. These four areas may require attention in terms of additional work experience or special practicum.

Lacey (1982) is among those who suggest a practicum in business and industry for students as well as course work in business and industrial psychology. Where such a practicum is unavailable, graduate students may be able to devise a program in a setting analogous to working in business and industry. For example, one graduate student in a counseling psychology program negotiated a year-long practicum at the university's Learning Resource Center, an agency which was frequently approached by individual faculty and academic departments for assistance on a wide variety of educational problems. The student consulted with the center's staff on issues of faculty stress and teacher–student conflict. For example, the student helped staff learn how to listen more effectively to faculty and also helped them teach faculty how to do the same with their students. As in business settings, he had to provide this expertise to individuals whose conceptual and language systems (e.g., psychological versus educational) were different from his.

Rippert-Davila (1985) compares consultation in business and industry to a journey in a new culture. To begin, the consultant must learn the language of business "by listening for key phrases, jargon, and acronyms in order to establish rapport and foster credibility" (p. 239). Again, this might also be accomplished by reading trade or company publications. She suggests that consultants be able to explain the rationale of their methods (e.g., collect data, share information, make decisions, implement program changes) and what specific outcomes those methods will produce (e.g., increased productivity or job satisfaction, decreased work stress). Also, unproductive stereotypes (e.g., that all multinational corporations aim to take advantage of developing countries) must be confronted by consultants in *themselves*.

Not all agree that special training is necessary for a mental health professional to work effectively as a consultant to business. Perloff (1982), for example, suggests that mental health consultants stick to what they do well—optimize personal decisions about work, leisure, and family—with the beneficial result of avoiding the retooling necessary for business work. Perloff believes that a huge marketplace already exists of workers who "are frustrated, who don't get along with supervisors, whose ideas are alien to the organization's" (p. 43). These workers are similar to the clients who typically walk through the office doors of many mental health professionals.

Finally, Wells (1983) discusses the details consultants should attend to before they begin a consulting assignment. Wells suggests that consultants should be prepared to provide potential employers with academic transcripts and references. Wells advises consultants to offer services at professional rates, avoid guaranteeing success or tying fees to outcomes, provide clients with time to make a decision about hiring consultants, and avoid selling one "pet system." Written proposals should be standardized and should precisely describe the program, identify responsibilities of both consultant and client, and set a schedule for completion of tasks. Fees and expenses should be specifically identified. Wells also advises a cancellation clause giving each party the right to terminate after appropriate notification.

Mental health consultants have also developed expectations concerning how consultees should perform. Kellogg (1984) interviewed 20 consultants to determine the factors that contribute to the development of successful client–consultant relationships. She found that the consultants valued clients' willingness to learn, intelligence, acceptance of feedback, willingness to take risks, and responsible follow-through on commitments. Consultants also believed it important to have a clear job description for themselves and the client, a respect for the consultant's competence by the client, and independent decision making by the client. Kellogg found that these consultants preferred to work with a contact person who had significant power in use of money for the consulting project and that they desired access to political information about the company for which they were consulting.

Kellogg's findings suggest that mental health consultants should develop preferences for the type of consulting situations and settings in which they will agree to work. In general, consultants should reconsider assignments where their clients appear uninvolved or uncommitted. It is possible that the consultation may produce harmful outcomes; for example, employees who complete a consultant's survey about the work environment may become demoralized when management fails to act on the findings. Saying no to inappropriate requests may be as important to a successful consulting career as effectively completing consultations.

SUMMARY

The opportunities for application of mental health principles in business and industry appear limited only by the imagination and willingness of consultants and consultees. Ideally, mental health consultants should be applying these principles to promote the development of human resources in business settings. This ideal seems to be rarely met, however, and it is the wise consultant who negotiates consulting conditions as well as fees before the consultation begins. For example, the consultant should be clear about protecting the confidentiality of employees who seek the help of a mental health professional.

It is apparent that in many settings consultants must be able to provide concrete evidence that their efforts substantially influence the company's productivity and profitability. A first step in this process may be to evaluate the outcomes of the consultation (see Chapter 9). Such evaluations document the effects of the consultation and when accompanied by cost-benefit and cost-effectiveness types of analysis, provide a rationale for the initiation and continuation of consultation efforts.

REFERENCES

APLIN, J. (1985). Business realities and organization consultation. *The Counseling Psychologist,* 13, 396–402.

BARKWAY, T., and KIRBY, N. (1983). The attitudes and opinions of Australian personnel management toward the contribution of industrial psychologists to human resource management. *Australian Psychologist,* 18 (3), 345–357.

BRILL, P., HERZBERG, J., and SPELLER, J. L. (1985). Employee Assistance Programs: An overview and suggested roles for psychiatrists. *Hospital and Community Psychiatry,* 36, 727–732.

BROWN, D. (1985). The preservice training and supervision of consultants. *The Counseling Psychologist,* 13, 410–425.

CAPLAN, G. (1970). *The theory and practice of mental health consultation.* New York: Basic Books.

CZANDER, W. M. (1986). *The application of social systems thinking to organizational consulting.* New York: University Press of America.

DEMUTH, N. M., YATES, B. T., and COATES, T. C. (1984). Psychologists as managers: Overcoming old guilts and accessing innovative pathways for enhanced skills. *Professional Psychology: Research and Practice,* 15 (5), 758–768.

DUSTIN, D., and BLOCHER, D. H. (1984). Theories and models of consultation. In Brown, S., and Lent, R. (eds.), *Handbook of counseling psychology.* New York: Wiley.

GAVIN, J. (1982). A "change of heart" is not enough. *The Counseling Psychologist,* 10 (3), 29–30.

GAVIN, J. F. (1977). Occupational mental health: Forces and trends. *Personnel Journal*, 56, 198–201.

GREINER, L. E., and METZGER, R. O. (1983). *Consulting to management.* Englewood Cliffs, NJ: Prentice Hall.

GROL, R., MOKKINK, H., SMITS, A., VAN EIJK, J., BEEK, M., MESKER, P., and MESKER-NEISTEN, J. (1985). Work satisfaction of general practitioners and the quality of patient care. *Family Practice*, 2, 128–135.

HIPPLE, J., and RAMSAY, A. (1985). Consultation through quality circles. *Journal of College Student Personnel*, 26, 556–558.

JACKSON, S. E. (1984). Organizational practices for preventing burnout. In A. S. Tehi and R. S. Schuler (eds.), *Handbook of organizational stress coping strategies.* Cambridge, MA: Ballinger.

KELLOGG, D. M. (1984). Contrasting successful and unsuccessful OD consultation relationships. *Group and Organization Studies*, 9, 151–176.

LACEY, D. W. (1982). Industrial counseling psychologists: The professional road not taken. *The Counseling Psychologist*, 10 (3), 49–51.

LEVY-LEBOYER, C. (1988). Success and failure in applying psychology. *American Psychologist*, 43, 779–785.

McCORMACK, I., and DeVORE, J. (1986). Survey-guided process consultation in a veterans administration medical center psychology service. *Professional Psychology: Research and Practice*, 17, 51–57.

MEIER, S. (1983). Toward a theory of burnout. *Human Relations*, 36, 899–910.

MINATOYA, L. Y. (1982). Comments on counseling psychology. *The Counseling Psychologist*, 10 (3), 27–28.

MOOS, R. H. (1981). *Work environment scale manual.* Palo Alto, CA: Consulting Psychologists Press.

MUCH, M. (1984). Getting the bugs out. *Industry Week*, May 14.

OSIPOW, S. H. (1982). Counseling psychology: Applications in the world of work. *The Counseling Psychologist*, 10 (3), 19–25.

OSKAMP, S. (1988). Non-traditional employment opportunities for applied psychologists. *American Psychologist*, 43, 484–485.

PERLOFF, R. (1982). The case for life satisfaction counseling as a critical role for the counseling psychologist in industry. *The Counseling Psychologist*, 10, 9–18.

RANDOLPH, D. L. (1985). *Microconsulting: Basic psychological consultation skills for helping professionals.* Johnson City, TN: Institute of Social Sciences and Arts, Inc.

RIDLEY, C. R., and HELLERVIK, L. W. (1982). Counseling psychology in the corporate environment. *The Counseling Psychologist*, 10 (3), 53–54.

RIPPERT-DAVILA, S. (1985). Cross-cultural training for business: A consultant's primer. *The Modern Language Journal*, 69, 238–246.

ROSKIES, E., SERAGANIAN, P., OSEASOHN, R., SMILGA, C., MARTIN, N., and HANLEY, J. A. (1989). Treatment of psychological stress responses in healthy Type A men. In R. W. J. Neufeld (ed.), *Advances in the investigation of psychological stress.* New York: John Wiley.

SIVER, E. W. (1983). The 10 commandments for choosing and using consultants. *Risk Management*, June, 64–74.

STARK, S., and ROMANS, S. (1982). Business and industry: How do you get there? *The Counseling Psychologist*, 10 (3), 45–47.

STERN, L. R. (1982). Response commentary on business and industry. *The Counseling Psychologist,* 10 (3), 37–38.

TOOMER, J. (1982). Counseling psychologists in business and industry. *The Counseling Psychologist,* 10, 9–18.

WELLS, R. G. (1983). What every manager should know about management consultants. *Personnel Journal,* February, 142–148.

WILBUR, C. S., and VERMILYEA, C. J. (1982). Some business advice to counseling psychologists. *The Counseling Psychologist,* 10 (3), 31–32.

YALOM, I. (1985). *The theory and practice of group psychotherapy.* New York: Basic Books.

ZIEGENFUSS, J. T., and LASKY, D. I. (1980). Evaluation and organizational development: A management-consulting approach. *Evaluation Review,* 4 (5), 665–676.

CHAPTER FIVE
CONSULTATION
IN MEDICAL SETTINGS

Despite significant obstacles, mental health consultants are increasingly finding their way into medical settings. The need for such consultation is obvious. Thompson and Peterson (1985) indicate that a high percentage of patients have emotional issues that constitute their primary problem or contribute significantly to their physical illness; untreated or unidentified emotional problems may interfere with medical care (Thompson and Peterson, 1985). For example, AIDS patients frequently develop organic mental disorders along with psychological stress and symptoms (Wolcott, Fawzy, and Pasnau, 1985).

Despite evidence of such need, many medical personnel exhibit considerable ambivalence about using mental health consultants. Surveys of physicians show that while many acknowledge the importance of emotional factors in physical illness, relatively few actually use a mental health consultant. One survey of actual consultation practices found that only 17 percent of the physicians used 50 percent of the consultation services (Daniels and Linn, 1984).

Partly as a result of this conflict between medicine and mental health, no systematic relationship is apparent between the skills of mental health consultants and the specific medical settings in which they are employed. Consultants are found in a wide variety of settings and with a wide variety of problems, including burn units (Ochitill, 1984), cancer treatment (Goldberg, Tull, Sullivan, Wallace, and Wool, 1984), internal medicine (Schubert, 1982), family practice (Oxman and Smith, 1982), chronic care facilities (Wasylenki and Harrison, 1981), pediatrics (Sherman, 1982), AIDS patients (Wolcott, Fawzy, and Pasnau), nursing homes (Sbordone and Sterman, 1983), health maintenance organizations (HMOs; Budman, 1985), and pain clinics (Hickling, Sison, and Holtz, 1985). What may be happening is that consultants are employed primarily in crisis situations or in settings where individual medical personnel are open to such consultation.

Gabinet and Friedson (1980) note that despite the overlap in training among psychiatrists, psychologists, and social workers, "as consultants to primary physicians, psychologists and social workers typically perform circumscribed functions" (p. 939). They suggest that mental health consultants accrue medical knowledge—"the mechanisms whereby physical disturbances can produce psychological changes and the psychological manifestations of organic dysfunction" (p. 944)—because such knowledge makes medical patients a new population which can potentially be helped by consultants. Such learning, they state, occurs best "through continuing on-the-job training" (p. 944).

This medical emphasis is also evident in sources of reports about mental health consultation in medical settings. Most of these reports discuss psychiatric consultation. References in the literature to nonpsychiatric consultants working in medical settings are relatively new and have increased just in the past decade (Gabinet and Friedson, 1980). However, many of the issues faced by psychiatric consultants in medical settings—resistance to consultation, for example—are also likely to be encountered by nonpsychiatric consultants.

This chapter will begin by reporting surveys on the use of and need for mental health consultants. In that way consultants may develop ideas about potential sites and services to pursue. Next, evidence regarding the effectiveness of mental health consultation is presented; consultants who evaluate their work in medical settings may find this information useful. The uneasy alliance between medicine and mental health is then explored in detail, providing some preparation for the obstacles consultants may face; consultants must understand this ambivalence in order to devise appropriate consulting strategies. Finally, examples of current mental health consultation in medical settings are described in detail.

SURVEYS OF USE AND NEED

When asked, many physicians indicate that they desire psychological consultation. For example, Schenkenberg, Peterson, Wood, and DaBell (1981) reported the results of a survey of 79 physicians in a VA medical center on their perceptions of the effectiveness of a psychological consultation service and the importance of psychological factors in medical disease. The service was provided by a staff psychologist and three psychology interns to medical and neurological wards. Schenkenberg and associates found a generally positive response to consultation services; the strongest support for psychological consultation was indicated for evaluating mental status and psychological disorders. Physicians gave their lowest ratings to the statement that "psychological factors are important in understanding the etiology of medical/neurological disease." Schenkenberg and associates reported that physicians expected consultants to be pleasant, compassionate, and possess a modest background in medical illness.

Liese (1986) conducted a similar survey in which he asked 80 physicians at a university medical center to rate 10 common medical problems according to the importance of psychological factors. The problems rated as having the largest psychological components were depression, alcoholism, obesity, and headaches; cancer, heart disease, and arthritis were rated as the problems with the lowest psychological influence. Liese also found that physicians were interested in treating the psychological components of illness themselves and that they would consult psychiatrists, psychologists, and social workers on an equal basis.

Both Schenkenberg and colleagues and Liese note that their surveys may not be representative of physicians' responses at other settings. Of particular note is that the physicians worked in a VA medical center and a university medical center, sites where physicians are more likely to have routine contact with mental health professionals.

To provide details about the use of mental health consultants, Daniels and Linn (1984) observed the use of a psychiatrist in a primary care medical center. They recorded 217 encounters with 63 service providers (primarily physicians and nurses). Daniels and Linn found that only 21 percent of the encounters involved seeing a patient, that most consultation occurred in an unplanned fashion, and that initial reasons for consultation often changed over the course of the consult. Medical personnel most often requested help about nondrug treatments, psychological referral sources, evaluations of patients, and exploring caregivers' feelings about patients. Most of the requests for consultation came from a relatively small group of persons: only 17 percent of the 63 providers requested 50 percent of the consults.

Wasylenki and Harrison (1981) reported a study of consultation practices in a chronic-care hospital. They recorded data on 70 consultations over a two-year period. Although 60 percent of requests were for depression, only 9 percent eventually received a diagnosis of affective disorder. About half of the patients seen were experiencing difficulty adapting to chronic disabling illnesses. Wasylenki and Harrison suggest that part of the process of adjusting to such illnesses involves a grief process wherein anxiety, anger, and sadness must be expressed. The important role a mental health consultant could play in facilitating such processes is obvious. They suggest that the goal of many consultations should be to reduce the number of drugs a patient consumes and that treatment should focus on interpersonal and milieu approaches.

Taylor and Doody (1979) discuss mental health consultations as they occurred over a five-year period in a general hospital. Sixty-five percent of referrals came from medical services, twice the rate from surgical services. Referral requests came most frequently for diagnosis and for evaluation of depression; other high-frequency requests centered on behavior management problems and suicide. Taylor and Doody note that the explicit reasons for consultation often differ from the actual problem. That is, a request to evaluate a difficult patient may actually lead the consultant to undertake work with conflict within the staff or between the doctor and patient.

Craig (1982) studied 308 actual consultations in a university hospital and found that the majority of referrals requested specific help with diagnosis and treatment. Craig notes that despite the high percentage of persons with psychological problems who see physicians, estimates range from only 1 to 10 percent for the number of these patients who physicians actually refer for emotional help. Craig's one-year study of consultations found that most of the requests involved diagnosis, depression, suicide, and alcohol. He also found that twice as many women were referred as men and that the elderly had low rates of referral. Patients themselves seldom requested a referral.

Gabinet and Friedson (1981) note a study by Billowitz and Friedson (1978) which found that nonpsychiatric physicians followed about two-thirds of the mental health consultants' recommendations and four-fifths of the recommendations for psychotropic medication. Interestingly, acceptance of mental health consultants' recommendations were equal to those of other consultants at the hospital.

Thompson and Peterson (1985) note that although estimates placed the number of persons with mental disorders at 15 percent of the U.S. population, only 20 percent of that group are seen by mental health specialists. Primary care physicians constitute the group most likely to see and treat persons with psychological disturbances. Thompson and Peterson's review of research indicates that physicians perform poorly in detecting psychological problems in their patients. These studies found that residents and physicians typically *miss* 50 to 90 percent of patients' psychological issues. Consequently, consultants may be called upon to train physicians in the diagnosis, treatment, and referral of psychological difficulties. Such training may involve suicide assessment and psychological aspects of the physician–patient relationship.

At a children's medical center, Rivara and Wasserman (1984) studied differences between a ward where a staff child psychiatrist routinely participated in daily teaching rounds to a ward without a child psychiatrist. Following a one-month period of such consultation, Rivara and Wasserman examined residents' daily progress notes and found no differences between wards on the overall proportion of psychosocial notes recorded or the quality of those notes. In total, only 18 percent of the notes discussed psychosocial aspects of the patient. Rivara and Wasserman explained their findings by suggesting that residents perceive physicians as role models primarily interested in the biomedical aspects of patients; psychosocial aspects, therefore, should be relegated to other health care professionals. In this study, then, use of a consultant did not increase residents' interest in or performance of psychosocial assessment but simply confirmed that such issues are in the realm of other personnel.

Stabler and Mesibov (1984) reviewed the roles of pediatric and health psychologists in health care settings. They surveyed 686 psychologists and found that two-thirds had their graduate training in the area of clinical psychology. Both pediatric and health psychologists spent about a third of their time doing treatment. Pediatric psychologists (child-clinical) also spent considerable time in diagnostic testing. Both groups reported problems because of "physicians' lack of knowledge concerning both psychological issues and ways in which psychologists can be utilized" (p. 147). When considering the goals of a consultant, however, changing physicians' attitudes was considered relatively unimportant by the survey respondents. Highly ranked goals were the transmission of technical or clinical information and service delivery.

Hengeveld and Rooymans (1983) reviewed the literature on mental health consultation with medical *staff* and found that a relatively small percentage of all consultations (about 10 percent on average) had to do with staff problems. They studied 313 consultations over a 14-month period carried out at a university hospital. About one-third of the consultations contained some indication of staff difficulties. They found, however, that consultants tended not to overtly approach staff members about their difficulties, ostensibly because the staff problem was judged not harmful or difficult to assess. Staff seemed to experience the most difficulty working with patients experiencing a negative reaction to their illness as opposed to a formal psychological disorder. One might expect, then, for staff to request consultations when patients' psychological difficulties are relatively unexpected (as in the case of a patient who experiences depression and withdrawal during a period of prolonged hospitalization) as compared to patients' whose primary difficulties are clearly psychological in nature (such as with a schizophrenic). In addition, Hengeveld and Rooymans found that the number of staff problems on surgical wards exceeded that of medical wards. They concluded that the need for staff consultation is relatively small and that such consultation should primarily be directed at the nursing staff on surgical wards, the initiators of many mental health consultations.

Hickling, Sison, and Holtz (1985) surveyed psychologists in multi-disciplinary pain clinics in the United States to determine their roles. Psychological factors like expectations, anxiety, and suggestion affect the experience of pain (Hickling, Sison, and Holtz, 1985). They found that psychologists in these settings spent about equal amounts of time functioning as therapists and evaluators. Behaviorally oriented interventions, such as relaxation and operant conditioning, are most often employed along with assessment devices such as the MMPI.

Budman (1985) reports that health maintenance organizations (HMOs) are growing rapidly across the United States and usually offer at least brief evaluative or crisis intervention services. Budman cited previous research indicating that between 50 and 80 percent of the general population seen in primary outpatient medical care settings have noticeable psychological problems. Initial data from several HMOs indicate that similarly high incidences of mental health problems are likely to be presented by patients in these new health care settings. Services provided by HMOs initially centered on traditional psychotherapy but over time have evolved to include smoking cessation, stress management, and pain control (Budman, 1985).

As Barsky and Brown (1982) note, patients are partners in the care process, carrying out the treatment, monitoring their status, deciding when to consult the physician, coping with disability, and practicing health maintenance. The researchers' study of mental health consultations suggests that consultants should work with the physician, instead of the patient, to avoid implying physician failure or incompetence. Principal problems for which consultation was requested included functional somatic complaints, noncompliance with medical recommendations, depression, psychosis, and alcoholism. Barsky and Brown noted that physicians tend to underestimate the efficacy of psychological procedures like support and active listening.

Sherman's (1982) examples of emergency consultation requests included aggressive children, problems with parents, diagnostic dilemmas, a request to discharge the next day, and the sudden involvement of an important person. She cited a study by Karasu that indicated that physicians most value consultants' direct intervention with patients and families. Physicians least valued direct intervention with staff such as teaching interviewing techniques, resolving conflicts among ward staff, helping staff deal with stress, and helping staff deal with their reactions to individual patients. Thus, physicians may be more interested in having consultants directly intervene with (troublesome?) patients than with altering physicians' skills and behaviors.

EFFECTIVENESS OF MENTAL HEALTH CONSULTATION

Although not without controversy, substantial evidence exists to suggest that emotional disturbances and physical illness are related and that attending to mental health ultimately benefits physical health (McKegney and Beckhardt, 1982). For example, Budman (1985) notes that most observers now conclude that psychotherapy reduces medical costs, although that effect seems to occur mainly with persons who limit their use of psychotherapy services to less than eight visits. A brief review is provided below.

Cummings (1977) discussed the mental health and medicine link while summarizing the debate about whether a national health insurance system should include a mental health component. Physical illness, Cummings wrote, is the result of problems of living: "The way we live, eat, drink, smoke, compete and pollute relate inevitably to strokes, heart attacks, cancer, obesity, malnutrition, paralysis, cirrhosis, migraine, suicide, and asthma, to list only a few" (p. 713). Because of the enormous costs, Cummings indicates that it is unlikely that any open-ended psychotherapy benefit will be available under national health insurance. Yet when therapy is provided as part of a comprehensive health system, "the costs of providing the benefit are more than offset by the savings in medical utilization" (p. 717). Active, brief psychotherapy may be the most effective in terms of cost and therapeutic benefits. Examining data from an HMO, Follette and Cummings (1967) found that persons in emotional distress were significantly high users of both inpatient and outpatient medical treatment. They also discovered that significant declines in medical care occurred with persons who received (even brief) psychotherapy.

Robson, France, and Bland (1984) compared a group of patients in a medical center who had access to a psychological consultant to a group who did not. The treatment group had 229 patients, while 200 persons constituted the control group; 72 percent of the subjects were female, and average age was 33 years. The treatment group had higher self-ratings of satisfactory outcome, fewer number of doctor visits, and lower overall drug costs.

Mumford, Schlesinger, Glass, Patrick, and Cuerdon (1984) presented a meta-analysis examining the cost-offset effects of outpatient mental health treatment. They reviewed 58 studies and found that 85 percent reported a decrease in medical utilization following psychotherapy. Previous research indicated that cost benefits occur after about six psychotherapy visits. Older patients showed more reduction in medical services following therapy, and reduction appeared largely in inpatient, not outpatient, costs.

Mitchell and Thompson (1985) suggest that researchers might best be able to demonstrate benefits of psychological intervention on such physical problems as "cardiovascular diseases, respiratory diseases such as asthma and COPD, diabetes, hypertension, and other illnesses in which there is a strong psychosomatic component" (p. 67). Schlesinger and colleagues report that cost savings related to medical service utilization may not appear until at least six months of treatment or until treatment ends. Such savings, however, seem to persist.

Freeman and Button (1984) observed the operation of a clinical psychological service in a medical center over a six-year period. A general decrease occurred in the use of psychotropic drugs and consultation rates for psychosocial problems across the whole medical center. From their reading of the practice data, Freeman and Button argue that the natural history of most psychological problems is one of crisis and natural remission, and in such a sequence a therapist is unlikely to make significant change. Thus, they conclude that the impact of a psychologist offering weekly sessions is small and precludes the introduction of the psychologist into the primary care team. They argue that the consultant can play an educational role, however, assisting physicians to learn about psychotherapeutic alternatives to psychotropic medications.

EXAMPLES

Teaching

Daniels and Shinn (1984) provide an example of teaching a first-year medical resident to attend to psychological cues in patients with physical symptoms. The resident requested assistance in evaluating a female patient for antidepressants. The woman had a chronic cardiac condition, had been repeatedly hospitalized, and had a long-term poor prognosis. On a recent admission she appeared tired and apathetic. Discussion with the patient indicated that she was experiencing sadness and grief about her loss of function and life. Working with the consultant, the resident then decided to schedule several short counseling sessions to allow her to ventilate feelings. He also decided that drugs were not appropriate at that time.

Thompson and Peterson (1984) propose that consultants educate physicians about the use of questionnaires to quickly and effectively screen for emotional problems and provide data for follow-up questions. They suggest that physicians be introduced to questionnaires such as the Beck Depression Inventory. Other tools which might be of benefit in screening include brief interviews to address questions about stress and social support.

Assessment

As noted in the surveys reported above, medical personnel frequently ask consultants to provide assessment services. However, medical personnel often do not realize that psychological assessments differ from typical medical laboratory tests. Daniels and Linn (1984) found that most medical providers initially had a single question but that multiple issues arose as the consultation continued. They suggest that "providers seemed unable to formulate independently the specific kind of help they needed and therefore initially approached the consultant with a request that was only remotely related to the consultation that resulted" (p. 201). This process contrasts with that of traditional psychological assessment in which assessors must first possess a clear question before they can proceed to properly select, administer, and interpret psychological tests (Matarazzo, 1987). For example, in one hospital it was common for the consultant to receive testing requests from physicians such as "Tell me what's the matter with her" or "Give him a Rorschach." In these cases it became clear that the physicians were applying their understanding of medical test use (e.g., give blood tests and see what turns up) to psychological and intellectual assessment. More appropriate questions (Davis, personal communication, December 13, 1988) would have been "Is the patient psychotic?" or "How depressed is this patient?" The potential conflict between caregivers' ambiguity about what help they need and consultants' need to have a clearly defined problem suggests that consultants must (1) be patient and (2) consider problem formulation and teaching about the problem area as crucial, initial aspects of the consultation process.

Cancer Patients

Koocher and associates (1979) describe the successful implementation of mental health consultation with cancer patients. Working together as a three-person consulting team, they began leading weekly psychological rounds on the unit. Their work now included counseling with families as well as individual patients, hypnosis and relaxation for problems with medication and needles, and neuropsychological assessment for leukemic children who underwent central nervous system irradiation. Koocher and associates also provided weekly teaching seminars on topics like psychological aspects of childhood cancer. As evidence of the facility's support for psychological consultation, Koocher et al. noted that two half-time positions continued to be funded despite a substantial number of service hours that were not billable to third-party payment.

Koocher et al. (1979) reported an example of an 11-year-old with leukemia who became extremely anxious about intravenous infusions and bone marrow biopsies, two frequently required procedures. He became hysterical before any procedure that involved a needle. The consultants taught the patient self-hypnosis and relaxation techniques in daily 40-minute sessions over a 2-week period. The consultant initially stayed with him during treatment procedures. The patient reported that he still experienced some pain but was less anxious and better tolerated the procedures.

He also talked about the anger and frustration he felt as a result of the treatment. The consultant decreased the number of sessions as the patient felt better and became an outpatient.

Interpersonal Problems

Selzer (1981) describes various methods of consulting around staff interpersonal problems. For example, Selzer suggests that staff may attempt to trick the consultant into punishing an important patient or a staff member who has political influence in the medical setting. Struggles may be going on among a unit's members, against the hospital administration, or with a patient's family. These struggles may be elicited by attempts at limit setting, discharge or transfer, or change in medication. By recognizing staff pressure, the consultant can explore with staff why they want the consultant to take sides.

Selzer suggests that the consultant attend to her or his own reactions to the group process. A good opportunity to do this occurs during case conference when the consultant may bring to life the hidden agendas of the conference. The case conference may reveal the covert dynamics of the treatment setting. As an example, Selzer described how the new members of a medical unit, which had never before employed electroshock treatment (ECT), began to discuss ECT treatment for a patient. Selzer suggests that discussion of this treatment approach was an indirect way of challenging the unit's old authority.

Selzer indicates that if the consultant is hired by the administration, staff may redirect their anger at the consultant. Similarly, if the consultant holds an important administrative position within the hospital, a dual role develops and it is difficult for staff to trust the consultant. Another difficulty can arise if patients and staff see the consultant as omnipotent. They begin to look for answers for which there are no clear-cut solutions and are surprised to discover that considerable differences of opinion exist.

Difficult Patients

Tarnow and Gutstein (1982) describe a patient in an intensive care unit whose severe temper tantrums, which occurred after minor provocations, disrupted staff. Half of the staff desired to get rid of this patient while the other half wanted treatment. In this case the consultant helped the staff to reinforce to a moderate degree the maintenance of rules and roles. The staff learned to encourage flexibility and growth in the patient while maintaining the patient's affect within manageable limits.

Gabinet and Friedson (1981) note that young male accident victims may find it difficult to endure immobilization in casts and traction over an extended period. After these patients feel well for a few days, they begin to become overloaded with physical energy. Gabinet and Friedson suggest that this combination of immobilization and energy may result in anxiety, depression, and acting out behavior. Similar difficulties may arise with patients who experience chronic back pain with no physical causes. These patients, Gabinet and Friedson note, often demand extra care and medication. In response, the nursing staff may doubt the realness of their pain and resent their demands for relief. With immobilized patients and chronic back-pain patients, Gabinet and Friedson suggest that consultants help the staff be supportive and set limits.

General Practice

Weinman and Medlik (1985) describe the use of psychological consultants as educators of and skill-sharers with general practitioners. Working in a general practice setting enables one to switch the focus from medical illness to prevention and health education. Weinman and Medlik suggest that consultants at such settings can run counseling groups (including self-help groups) and classes for patients with problems like smoking, unassertiveness, bereavement, postnatal depression, stress, and eating disorders.

Weinman and Medlik (1985) suggest that general practitioners realize that much of their continuing education needs relate to psychological skills. Consultants can teach physicians how to make medical information comprehensible and to allow patients to discuss their problems. They describe a comprehensive course for physicians' problem solving and decision making which includes instruction about early confirmation biases of hypotheses. By deciding on diagnoses too soon, for example, physicians may not hear valuable information provided by patients.

Weinman and Medlik also outline a course to teach undergraduate medical students about the role of psychological factors in physical illness and about the prevalence of psychological problems in a general practice setting. This course includes teaching of basic counseling and interviewing skills. Evaluation of this course indicated that students displayed a greater ability to detect psychosocial influences compared to students who did not complete the course. They also describe an eight-week course designed to teach trainees, through the use of videotaped consultations, role play, seminars, and discussion, such skills as attending to nonverbal behavior, relaxation training, and assertiveness training.

Wright and Burns (1986) suggest that mental health care in primary care settings differs from traditional psychological service: more clients are seen, less time is spent with each, and clients are less severely disturbed. Short-term therapy with more developmental problems is the norm in such settings. They assert that training primary care physicians in interviewing skills and in targeting certain mental health problems can increase accurate identification of psychological issues.

AIDS

Organic mental disorders, stress, and psychological symptoms are frequently present in AIDS patients (Wolcott, Fawzy, and Pasnau, 1985). Wolcott and colleagues suggest that consultants may be useful in diagnosing and treating organic mental disorders, psychosocial and neuro-psychiatric aspects of AIDS, grief counseling, and health-care professional stress. Dementia, language disorders, and delirium appear to be relatively common features with AIDS. More important to the psychological consultant are problems such as depression, anxiety, crisis, loss of social support, and grieving. Friends and family of AIDS patients face a long period of providing physical and emotional support. Health care professionals may fear AIDS infection, hold negative attitudes towards AIDS patients, or experience emotional exhaustion after treatment with many AIDS patients.

Although AIDS is a unique disease, much of the psychological treatment employed with cancer and other terminally ill patients may be transferable to patients with the new disease. Persons who have just learned that they have AIDS may panic, and crisis intervention skills are then applicable (Dilley and Goldblum, 1987). Similarly, grief counseling—helping patients who are denying, angry, bargaining, depressed and, eventually, accepting of their illness and eventual death—may be useful with AIDS patients (Doubleday, 1987).

Chronic Care

Wasylenki and Harrison (1981) note that persons with serious illnesses may react to their diagnosis by regressing to such primitive defenses as denial and pseudoindependence. In the case of terminally ill patients who deny, they suggest that consultants confront the denial in a nurturant atmosphere in which sadness and anger are tolerated. Similarly, stroke patients may interpret their illness as punishment for sins and consequently feel guilty. Such patients, Wasylenki and Harrison maintain, have a fear of being left permanently crippled and experience loss of control when they compare their current situation to the past.

Nursing Homes

Another problem for which mental health consultants may be able to offer assistance concerns the high rate of turnover in nursing home staff. Such turnover costs the home money (e.g., in constantly training new employees), increases the workload on remaining staff, lowers patient care and staff productivity, and frustrates administrators who must continually hire new staff (Sbordone and Sterman, 1983).

Sbordone and Sterman (1983) reported on a 12-week program-centered consultation aimed at reducing staff turnover and improving morale at a 188-bed nursing home. They met "considerable suspicion and contempt" by the home's administrator and nursing director at initial sessions. Sbordone and Sterman spent time educating staff about the functions and purposes of consultation; they explained their method as a systems approach in which no one individual was to blame for problems of the home. Further meetings were held with staff to learn their frustrations about work. Difficulties included poor communication among staff (particularly among nursing aides who felt excluded from decision-making processes, even from offering their opinions), poor treatment of staff (e.g., calling nursing aids "kids"), difficult work with little or no reward, and frequent transfer of the top administrator to other homes (to the extent that staff could ignore any current administrator's decisions). The staff appeared to work primarily to avoid punishment, a condition Sbordone and Sterman attribute to a management style that attempted to control employee behavior through negative reinforcement.

Sbordone and Sterman reported an increased level of trust by the staff toward the consultants by the eighth week. Further work centered on improving communication among levels of staff and administrators and on methods of financially rewarding staff for desired behavior. Evaluation of the consultation by 50 randomly selected staff indicated improved morale and a willingness to participate in further staff meetings. Turnover rate declined by half during the consultation period (to 28 percent) and remained at comparable levels for the next nine months.

Burn Units

Ochitill (1984) noted studies which suggest that patients on burn units frequently have a history of psychological problems. Staff who work with these patients, Ochitill indicates, may also benefit from consultation because of the stresses associated with their work: patients' with disfigurement and death resulting from burns, the demanding behavior of some patients, and the difficulty of administering painful treatments, particularly to children. Psychological interventions to help burn patients in pain include explanations of treatment, cognitive strategies, and teaching of skills for pain management.

Ochitill reported an example of a 32-year-old man who was hostile to staff and resisted dressing changes. The staff regarded his behavior as an indication of character pathology. Upon interviewing the patient, the consultant learned that he was bothered by his reputation among the staff and felt helpless. The consultant shared the interview with staff. Staff members began to teach the patient about treatment, rewarded him when he acted on his own behalf, and looked for opportunities for him to assist in continuing care.

Obstetrics and Gynecology

Opposition to the paternalism and impersonal nature of modern medicine is especially prevalent in obstetrics and gynecology, Stotland (1985) suggests. The result is increased interest in self-help activities such as child-birth preparation classes. Stotland indicates that mental health consultations may be helpful for persons involved in such procedures as artificial insemination, hysterectomy, and fetuses with genetic risk.

Solyom (1981) proposes that mental health consultants work with staff of agencies that provide infant care. She suggests that lengthy separations from the mother for very young children, changing staff, and inconsistent caretaking attitudes are factors which have potential to harm infants. Mental health professionals could help, Solyom indicates, by meeting weekly with the caregiver staff for consultation and teaching caregivers how to perform systematic observations of infants' affect and interpersonal relationships. Consultants could prevent mental health difficulties if they help the staff to become "able to accurately perceive, empathically understand, and appropriately and flexibly respond to the child's communications" (p. 192).

Solyom also notes that consultants could assist parents who are having difficulty raising their children, such as unwed teenage mothers. She suggests that the consultant model basic listening skills and empathy for the staff who, in turn, model those skills and qualities to the parents. Staff's acquisition of this psychological knowledge may also increase their own personal growth, work satisfaction, and desire to stay on the job.

ISSUES

The information presented above offers an interesting paradox in the provision of mental health consulting in medical settings. On the one hand, the need for such consultation is apparent: attention to emotional issues seems to have positive effects on physical illness. At the same time, considerable resistance exists among medical personnel to use of mental health consultation. This ambivalence has its costs: in an era in which cost and accountability are becoming paramount, misdiagnosing psychological problems as physical illnesses rates as an expensive mistake.

As Koocher, Sourkes, and Keane (1979) note, the traditional medical model, which portrays emotional distress in terms of disease or illness, creates problems for the mental health consultant. With a medical consultation, the physician typically calls in a specialist who examines the record and the patient, performs tests, and then provides information to the physician. Koocher and associates suggest that with psychological issues, it is much more difficult for the consultant to specify the problem's origins, symptoms, and most effective treatment approach. Tarnow and Gutstein (1982) note the stress typically experienced by psychiatrists working as consultants in medical settings. They review research which employs terms like "frustrating," "hopelessness," and "demoralizing" to describe how such consultants feel upon meeting continual resistance to their work.

If it is difficult for mental health consultants to work with emotional issues, then it is doubly so for many medical personnel. Koocher and associates (1979) provide an example of a 17-year-old male patient who developed a bone tumor requiring an amputation. Despite radiation therapy and chemotherapy, the tumor spread to the spinal cord. The patient experienced increasing levels of physical disability and began to withdraw. Staff did not request a consult until he had an overt anxiety attack, rocking in bed and threatening to jump out the window. Koocher and associates suggest that most consults occur only with crisis situations like this one.

Koocher et al. (1979) also found that the nursing staff at their pediatric oncology unit was eager to have regular access to mental health consultation. As a result, a psychologist arranged to be at the unit daily at a regularly scheduled time. Over the following months the staff moved away from crisis consultations and requested more assistance for prevention. In addition, staff became more sophisticated in their referrals (e.g., differentiating between parents who needed direct contact with the consultant or who required only indirect consultation with the staff).

Gabinet and Friedson (1981) report that evidence exists to suggest that physicians do not want to learn about psychosocial factors of their patients or patient–staff interactions. They review speculations about physicians' apparent disinterest, including overwork, preoccupation with medical problems, and feelings of inadequacy. Gabinet and Friedson's experience at a major urban hospital was that nurses and social workers make most of the referrals for mental health consultation. Thompson and Peterson (1984) suggest that physicians avoid psychological issues because of a lack of time, fear that they are invading patients' privacy, difficulty in locating and maintaining referral sources, and lack of training.

Goleman (1988) reviews research which suggests that most physicians lack interviewing skills. Physicians tend to ignore patients' sense of their illness while dominating the interview with questions designed to produce a medical diagnosis. Good interviews, according to Goleman, should include patients' explanations of their personal concerns as well as their physical complaints. Collaboration between patient and physician in diagnosis and treatment may lead to greater compliance in taking drugs and following recommendations and increased patient satisfaction. Goleman also reported on another study of 336 doctor–patient encounters which found that physicians frequently underestimated patients' desire for information and overestimated how much information they had shared. This lack of communication may lead to such difficulties as patients' misunderstanding of medication advice.

Some evidence exists to support the idea that stress in physicians' work is at least partially responsible for lack of attention to psychosocial factors. Grol, Mokkink, Smits, Van Eijk, Beek, Mesker, and Mesker-Niesten (1985) studied the work satisfaction of 57 general practitioners and its relation to the quality of patient care. They found that physicians who felt more positive about work paid more attention to the psychosocial aspect of patients' complaints and were generally more open to patients. More negative feelings about work, assessed in terms of physicians' experience of frustration, lack of time, and stress, correlated with giving little explanation to patients and a high prescription rate. Grol and colleagues suggest that "Doctors are not as a rule open about the tensions and difficulties they experience in their work" (p. 134). They recommend that physicians pay more attention to their feelings about work during training and continuing education.

Budman (1985) also discusses physicians' difficulties in addressing patients' mental health problems. He cites studies indicating that (1) physicians frequently misdiagnose depression as anxiety and subsequently prescribe the wrong medication; (2) 71 to 91 percent of patients who committed suicide had recently seen a physician, most of whom missed suicidal gestures made by these patients; and (3) over half of patients who committed suicide by overdose had received a prescription for the medication from their physician.

Sbordone and Sterman (1983) note that staff in nursing homes typically have little knowledge of psychological aspects of patient care. In addition, such staff may have little tolerance for emotional problems. Many of the problems associated with physicians in medical settings appear to be present in nursing homes. For example, high percentages of patients possess psychological difficulties which go unrecognized and untreated. Sbordone and Sterman suggest that mental health consultants may be able to help nursing home staff by providing training about psychological issues. However, implementation of such treatment is often resisted by staff and administrators and may be discontinued beyond its experimental period.

Discussing the relationship between psychiatrists and other medical personnel, Fink (1985) suggests that physicians must accept "what psychiatry is and what it can do" (p. 205). Fink's comment about conflicts between psychiatric and medical models applies to mental health consultation in general. Such consultation is more likely to be successful with medical personnel who understand how emotions can cause, maintain, and add to physical illness. Fink, however, maintains that previous education programs designed to assist physicians in learning about emotional factors in order to treat such problems as depression or sexual difficulties have failed. On the other hand, Wright and Burns (1986) claim that training physicians in interviewing skills and in targeting certain mental health problems has been demonstrated to increase accurate identification of psychological issues. Fink (1985) suggests that physicians have no real motivation to increase the time spent talking to their patients or to decrease the use of psychotropic medications. Part of the problem, Fink suggests, is that most physicians receive only a few courses and a brief six- to eight-week training experience in psychiatry.

Fink's (1985) solution to these difficulties is to revive the mind–body connection as "a scientific, biologic concept" (p. 206). He cites recent research demonstrating links between stress and the immune system and between good mental and physical health. Fink would, however, place the role of mental health consultation solely in the hands of psychiatrists: "the responsibility for reeducating primary care trainees and graduates about the mind and its functioning, about behavioral abnormalities, as well as about interviewing and communication skills, counseling patients, and the doctor–patient relationship really belongs to psychiatry" (p. 208).

Discussing problems in medical education, Korr (1987) refers to the "missing person" syndrome in which organs or technology are emphasized to the exclusion of psychosocial factors and the neglect of health promotion and disease prevention. Korr also criticizes the reification of disease (i.e., the view that the disease is different and apart from the patient): "However we think and talk about diseases, the fact is that nobody has ever seen one" (p. 6). Korr maintains that that medical model overlooks inherent healing mechanisms and the fact that it is the patient who gets well.

Dana and May (1986) note that psychiatrists have moved away from previous interests in psychoanalysis and community mental health towards a remedicalization of the field in terms of psychopharmacology and psychopathology. They cite Kupers (1981) as saying psychiatry's problems lie in "the profession's snobbishness, reliance on stultifying medication, and involuntary hospitalization."

Shectman and Harty (1982) note the current emphasis on biological etiology and psychopharmacology. Such a focus may be derived from a desire to portray psychological difficulty as an illness only treatable with medicine and to exclude nonphysician mental health workers from patient care. On the other hand, there is some suggestion that at least part of the medical field is moving away from the disease model. Dana and May (1986) suggest that medicine is becoming increasingly "demythologized" as individuals take more responsibility for their own health. Part of this process, they suggest, should entail increased attention to concerns about the physician–patient relationship. Dana and May quote former Surgeon General Jules Richmond (1979) as suggesting that attention to such factors as lifestyle and self-care may have greater impact on health status than changes in the medical services.

Shectman and Harty (1982) also discuss how conflicts between psychiatrists and psychologists can be damaging to patients. Such conflicts are certainly not limited to psychiatrists and psychologists. Conflict exists between many mental health professions over overlap of roles. If carried to extremes, such conflict can prevent optimal patient care. Differences between psychiatrists, psychologists, social workers, and counselors tend to be chiefly historical. Each profession began and evolved in different contexts, and it is this history, not necessarily the skills, training, and interest of individual practitioners, which often determines what tasks a mental health professional is asked or allowed to perform. For example, the psychiatric profession developed from the influence of Sigmund Freud and reflects his status as a physician and his development of psychoanalytic treatment. Psychologists can trace their professional development to the use of personality and vocational testing in World War II. Despite these different historical trends, considerable overlap in interests and competencies exist among the mental health professions. Thus, some psychologists provide psychoanalytic psychotherapy, while some psychiatrists administer psychological interviews and tests.

One of the effects of this lack of differentiation among fields is that stiff competition can exist for provision of services in medical settings where all four mental health professions are employed. Thus, a psychologist who has been hired by physicians to consult about patient–staff interaction may encounter resistance on a unit where social workers usually teach medical residents the basics of communication skills. Similarly, a psychiatrist who consults by teaching a nurse how to help an anxious patient relax may be resented by a psychologist whose training includes relaxation therapy but who primarily provides psychological assessment on the unit. Psychological consultants may be wise to assess the availability of mental health workers with similar competencies when they agree to work in medical settings. If other professionals are present with needed skills, the consultant should attempt to engage those professionals as a team or educate administrators about the resources they have available to continue services once the consultation concludes.

Allen (1981) notes that psychologists who consult with psychiatrists about diagnosis may end up in a competition to determine which label is correct. Allen suggests that psychologists in such consultation determine in advance what is expected of them regarding diagnosis. If testing is requested, Allen suggests that assessment data relevant to diagnosis be combined with historical data recovered through a clinical interview.

Goldberg, Tull, Sullivan, Wallace, and Wool (1984) attempt to describe the different contributions of psychiatrists, psychologists, social workers, and nurses to the practice of psychosocial oncology. Goldberg and associates maintain that psychiatrists' strengths lie in their ability to provide differential diagnosis, including the ability to determine if biomedical factors are producing psychological symptoms. They suggest that psychologists with a behavioral medicine background may provide therapy to aid patients with the stress and loss of control common with cancer treatment; psychologists may also provide neuropsychological assessment and skills in research methodology. Nursing staff may best be able to provide a liaison with the staff providing direct care to the patient, while social workers may best deliver information about the patients' social network, community resources, and financial aspects of health care.

Combining these different professions can provide an effective multidisciplinary team, Goldberg and associates (1984) maintain. They suggest that such a team be drawn from a department of psychiatry so that problems with salary support, lack of clinical accountability, and nonattendance at departmental meetings can be avoided. Goldberg et al. also suggest that such a team cannot be successful unless each member respects "each professional's autonomous judgement and contribution" (p. 20). Nonpsychiatrists should learn to speak the language of the physician as well as their own disciplines and be aware of psychological problems that actually have physiological causes. Even while attempting to differentiate among the professions, Goldberg et al. note the large overlap and say that it "is currently very controversial as to whether any single disciple [*sic*] can lay claim to unique expertise in psychotherapy" (p. 22).

As an example of strategies for working in a politically charged atmosphere, Schubert (1982) suggests that mental health consultants get to know consultees personally and make suggestions in a tentative fashion. The consultant should accept all consultation requests and avoid being hesitant or critical of physicians making the referral. Schubert further suggests that when brief or nonspecific requests occur, consultants should elicit more specific information by asking if there is an interest in psychosocial history, patient dynamics, diagnosis, or prognosis. Brief explanations of the consultant's recommendations may be useful along with references to relevant literature.

SUMMARY

The examples of mental health consultation described above run the gamut of medical service settings. Consultants would seem to be hindered only by their ingenuity in identifying potential sites and services. Research, moreover, has demonstrated both the need for and usefulness of mental health consultation. Nevertheless, nonpsychiatric consultants are only now beginning to make significant inroads into medicine. Given the history and depth of conflict between the medical and mental health professions, further progress in integrating emotional consultation into medical practice is likely to be slow but steady.

REFERENCES

ALLEN, J. G. (1981). The clinical psychologist as a diagnostic consultant. *Bulletin of the Menninger Clinic*, 45 (3), 247–258.

BARSKY, A. J., and BROWN, H. N. (1982). Psychiatric teaching and consultation in a primary care clinic. *Psychosomatics*, 23 (9), 908–921.

BUDMAN, S. H. (1985). Psychotherapeutic services in the HMO: Zen and the art of mental health maintenance. *Professional Psychology: Research and Practice*, 16 (6), 798–809.

CRAIG, T. J. (1982). An epidemiologic study of a psychiatric liaison service. *General Hospital Psychiatry*, 4, 131–137.

CUMMINGS, N. A. (1977). The anatomy of psychotherapy under national health insurance. *American Psychologist*, 32, 711–718.

DANA, R. H., and MAY, W. T. (1986). Health care megatrends and health psychology. *Professional Psychology: Research and Practice*, 17 (3), 251–255.

DANIELS, M. L., and LINN, L. S. (1984). Psychiatric consultation in a medical clinic: What do medical providers want? *General Hospital Psychiatry*, 6, 196–202.

DILLEY, J., and GOLDBLUM, P. (1987). AIDS and mental health. In V. Gong and N. Rudnick (eds.), *AIDS facts and issues*. New Brunswick, NJ: Rutgers University Press.

DOUBLEDAY, W. (1987). Death, dying, and AIDS. In V. Gong and N. Rudnick (eds.), *AIDS facts and issues*. New Brunswick, NJ: Rutgers University Press.

FINK, P. J. (1985). Psychiatry and primary care: Can a working relationship develop? *General Hospital Psychiatry*, 7, 205–209.

FOLLETTE, W. T., and CUMMINGS, N. A. (1967). Psychiatric service and medical utilization in a prepaid health plan setting. *Medical Care*, 5, 25–35.

FREEMAN, G. K., and BUTTON, E. J. (1984). The clinical psychologist in general practice: A six-year study of consulting patterns for psychosocial problems. *Journal of the Royal College of General Practitioners*, 34, 377–389.

GABINET, L., and FRIEDSON, W. (1981). The impact of ward dynamics on psychiatric consultation and liaison. *Comprehensive Psychiatry*, 22 (6), 603–611.

GABINET, L., and FRIEDSON, W. (1980). The psychologist as front-line mental health consultant in a general hospital. *Professional Psychology*, 11, 939–945.

GOLDBERG, R. J., TULL, R., SULLIVAN, N., WALLACE, S., and WOOL, M. (1984). Defining discipline roles in consultation psychiatry: The multidisciplinary team approach to psychosocial oncology. *General Hospital Psychiatry*, 6, 17–23.

GOLEMAN, D. (1988). Physicians may bungle key part of treatment: The medical interview. *The New York Times*, January 21, p. B10.

GROL, R., MOKKINK, H., SMITS, A., VAN EIJK, J., BEEK, M., MESKER, P., and MESKER-

NIESTEN, J. (1985). Work satisfaction of general practitioners and the quality of patient care. *Family Practice,* 2, 128–135.

HENGEVELD, M. W., and ROOYMANS, H. G. (1983). The relevance of a staff-oriented approach in consultation psychiatry: A preliminary study. *General Hospital Psychiatry,* 5, 259–264.

HICKLING, E. J., SISON, G. F., and HOLTZ, J. L. (1985). Role of psychologists in multidisciplinary pain clinics: A national survey. *Professional Psychology: Research and Practice,* 16 (6), 868–880.

KOOCHER, G. P., SOURKES, B. M., and KEANE, W. M. (1979). Pediatric oncology consultations: A generalizable model for medical settings. *Professional Psychology,* August, 467–474.

KORR, I. (1987). Medical education: The resistance to change. *Advances,* 4, 5–10.

LIESE, B. S. (1986). Physicians' perceptions of the role of psychology in medicine. *Professional Psychology: Research and Practice,* 17 (3), 276–277.

MCKEGNEY, F. P., and BECKHARDT, R. M. (1982). Evaluative research in consultation–liaison psychiatry: Review of the literature: 1970–1981. *General Hospital Psychiatry,* 4, 197–218.

MITCHELL, W. D., and THOMPSON, T. L. (1985). Some methodological issues in consultation–liaison psychiatry research. *General Hospital Psychiatry,* 7, 66–72.

MUMFORD, E., SCHLESINGER, H., GLASS, G. V., PATRICK C., and CUERDON, T. (1984). A new look at evidence about reduced cost of medical utilization following mental health treatment. *American Journal of Psychiatry,* 141, 1145–1158.

OCHITILL, H. (1984). Psychiatric consultation to the burn unit: The psychiatrist's perspective. *Psychosomatics,* 25 (9), 689–701.

OXMAN, T. E., and SMITH, R. (1982). Consultation–liaison psychiatry within a family practice. *Social Psychology,* 17, 101–107.

RIVARA, F. P., and WASSERMAN, A. L. (1984). Teaching psychosocial issues to pediatric house officers. *Journal of Medical Education,* 59, 45–53.

ROBSON, M. H., FRANCE, R., and BLAND, M. (1984). Clinical psychologist in primary care: Controlled clinical and economic evaluation. *British Medical Journal,* 288, 1805–1808.

SBORDONE, R. J., and STERMAN, L. T. (1983). The psychologist as a consultant in a nursing home: Effect on staff morale and turnover. *Professional Psychology: Research and Practice,* 14 (2), 240–250.

SCHENKENBERG, T., PETERSON, L., WOOD, D., and DABELL, R. (1981). Psychological consultation/liaison in a medical and neurological setting: Physicians' appraisal. *Professional Psychology,* 12 (3), 309–317.

SCHUBERT, D. S. (1982). Psychiatric consultation to internal medicine: A psychiatrist's thoughts. *Psychosomatics,* 23 (8), 833–843.

SELZER, M. A. (1981). The role of the consultant in the case conference: Some neglected aspects. *Psychiatry,* 44, 60–68.

SHECTMAN, F., and HARTY, M. K. (1982). Mental health disciplines in conflict: The patient pays the price. *Bulletin of the Menninger Clinic,* 46 (5), 458–464.

SHERMAN, M. (1982). Communicating: A practical guide for the liaison psychiatrist. *Psychiatric Clinics of North America,* 5 (2), 271–281.

SOLYOM, A. E. (1981). Mental health consultant in infant day care: A new frontier of prevention. *Infant Mental Health Journal,* 2, 188–197.

STABLER, B., and MESIBOV, G. B. (1984). Role functions of pediatric and health psychologists in health care settings. *Professional Psychology: Research and Practice,* 15 (2), 142–151.

STOTLAND, N. L. (1985). Contemporary issues in obstetrics and gynecology for the consultation–liaison psychiatrist. *Hospital and Community Psychiatry,* 36 (10), 1102–1108.

TARNOW, J. D., and GUTSTEIN, S. E. (1982). Systemic consultation in a general hospital. *International Journal Psychiatry in Medicine,* 12 (3), 161–186.

TAYLOR, G., and DOODY, K. (1979). Psychiatric consultations in a Canadian general hospital. *Canadian Journal of Psychiatry,* 24, 717–723.

THOMPSON, T. L., and PETERSEN, J. L. (1985). Improving recognition of psychiatric disorders in a primary care practice. *Psychiatric Disorders,* 78 (8), 155–162.

WASYLENKI, D., and HARRISON, M. K. (1981). Consultation–liaison psychiatry in a chronic care hospital: The consultation function. *Canadian Journal of Psychiatry,* 26, 96–100.

WEINMAN, J., and MEDLIK, L. (1985). Sharing psychological skills in the general practice setting. *British Journal of Medical Psychology,* 58, 223–230.

WOLCOTT, D. L., FAWZY, F. I., and PASNAU, R. O. (1985). Acquired immune deficiency syndrome (AIDS) and consultation–liaison psychiatry. *General Hospital Psychiatry,* 7, 280–292.

WRIGHT, L., and BURNS, B. J. (1986). Primary mental health care: A "find" for psychology? *Professional Psychology: Research and Practice,* 17 (6), 560–564.

CHAPTER SIX
CONSULTING
WITH GROUPS

Consultation is a process of horizontal communication that fosters a peer relationship for the purpose of collaboration. It provides a setting where support for professional approaches are offered and creative thinking is developed. Consultation is a major vehicle for bringing needed knowledge and services to others. Group consultation is a method of offering this knowledge to larger numbers of people in settings that can enhance the learning process. Group consultation will be addressed in terms of group consultation goals, leading consultation groups, group consultation dynamics, stages of group consultation, issues, and the ethics of confidentiality. Consultation groups are subject to the principles of group dynamics (Brown, Wyne, Blackburn, and Powell, 1979). They closely resemble any group which has a specified task and tends to move through similar stages. Consequently, group consultation leaders must possess leadership skills that include understanding group dynamics and group developmental skills.

GROUP CONSULTATION GOALS

Clear communication about the purpose(s) of the group is important. The group consultation leader arrives at the goals in the process of the entry stage and in the development of the contract. In many cases the consultation group will resemble a task-oriented group, which needs to have its purposes for meeting defined and clarified. The written contract, developed in the entry stage, becomes a working contact. This contract is verbalized with the group members; it is expanded and defined in ways all members can understand and accept. If the group's purpose for meeting is specific, such as a group of teachers learning to deal with alcoholism or a group of counselors coping with early terminations, these purposes should be clearly stated. This is part of structuring the group and it is the primary responsibility of the group leader. Frustration develops in members when the purpose is not stated or when it gets changed without group consent.

Since this is a consulting group rather than a counseling group, it is important to establish that the group process will be a collaborative one. The collaborative experience involves the opportunity and ability to learn from one another. This approach, however, is not common in many institutional settings. For example, hospital settings do not promote horizontal communication. Hospitals, like so many other institutions, are hierarchical in organization. The communication process moves vertically reducing the opportunity for collaborative relating. Consequently, the collaborative approach may need to be learned before it can be trusted as a viable and safe approach. The consultant will need to spend time teaching, especially modeling, collaboration. Sbordone and Sterman (1983) describe the need for fostering good interpersonal communications among staff and between hierarchical levels. In some institutions this is prevented. Supervisory personnel control the more formal communication network, which encourages the development of an informal communication system. The outcome is often the alienation of two groups and sometimes passive-aggressive behaviors. The introduction of a collaborative approach and open communication will require careful presentation on the part of the consultant and time to learn this new style.

The group consultation leader can facilitate the collaborative approach by identifying the members' roles. Members need to be identified as having the capacity of contributing to the learning process collaboratively. They need to be encouraged to present problems for discussion and group feedback. This is likely to be difficult, especially for some members who may feel awkward or insecure. Insecure members require a highly supportive and reinforcing atmosphere. The leader can create an atmosphere in which all members will participate. Some group leaders address this concern by stating a guideline that all criticism is to be phrased in a constructive fashion. Other leaders will structure the group process so that the group proceeds without getting bogged down in ambivalences. For example, when the group consultation's purpose is case review, the leader can provide a format for presenting the case followed by guidelines for responses from the group. The format for presenting the case may simply include background data on the client, a history of the client's problem, a description of the problem to date, a statement about what kind of assistance the member wishes from the group, and any issues of a professional and/or personal nature which may be useful to address. When all members are familiar with the outline, attending to the case will be easier and the presenting consultee will likely be more organized. This approach will create a routine for the group. Routines allow group expectations to come together and be less divergent. The group can then proceed with a common direction; this lends itself to healthy development of the group process.

Maintaining proper focus on the purpose for the consultation rests in the hands of the leader. The leader needs to guide the group as it defines the reasons for its existence. In the early stages, the focus should be on common topics and concerns (Brown, Wyne, Blackburn, and Powell, 1979). The process is to be shared in a collaborative way by all members rather than dominated by one or a few. For example, when a group of social service workers from a family protection unit met to learn more about family dynamics and apply this to their cases, it was important that general examples be used which could apply to many if not all the members. Examples used by the group leader must include, not exclude, group members. In the same way, individual members need to be reminded of the shared purpose of the group and be encouraged to remain focused. The consultant wants to maintain the sense of purpose so that members do not lose interest and the group process does not get interrupted. Maintaining focus on the purpose can be a shared experience of group members but ultimately rests with the consultant.

LEADING CONSULTATION GROUPS

The group consultant needs skills which match those of the group counselor: understanding group process and group dynamics and knowing how to lead a group are all essential. Yet, they are not enough by themselves. The consultant must blend consulting and counseling in order to offer an effective group consultation. Thus, group consultation necessitates a greater variety of skills than individual consultation. This is often why group consultation is not provided and, when it is, problems often occur because of the limited knowledge of the consultant. If the consultant is not trained and skilled in group dynamics, the group approach is likely to be ineffective. In the following, group dynamics and the role of group members will be presented in conjunction with the group consultant's role as leader.

Leadership Role

In group settings, the consultant initially assumes the responsibility for organizing and leading the group. Some institutions will take the responsibility for planning; however, if this task is not filled by someone from within the institution the consultant, whether from inside or outside, needs to play the role of organizer. This is a critical part of the entry and contracting stages. Organizing a group consultation requires a good deal of time arranging meeting times, location for the group meetings, attendance, and approval for the group activity. Setting up a group consultation is best done by those within the institution, perhaps the administration, since it requires knowledge of the institution. For example, it can be difficult for an outside consultant to gain access to teachers' schedules in order to establish a teachers' consultation group. It is far more likely that the principal can arrange this and locate a room for this purpose. These tasks are more economically done by school staff than by an outside consultant. It is within the parameter of the consultant's role to suggest the school make these arrangements. The consultant is then free to coordinate the process and attend to other concerns. Coordination is assisted with good, clear communication channels.

Enlisting institutional personnel to arrange for the consultation group does not mean the task is insignificant. It is a very important aspect of the group experience. The time the consultees meet has a great deal to do with their attitude about the program. If they arrive tired, distraught, meeting at an inconvenient time because the schedule was hastily arranged, the chances are high that they begin with concerns external to the planned agenda. Meeting at a time convenient to all is an important beginning for a collaborative experience. It is also true that the location of the consultation group is worth someone's attention. Consultees in schools, for example, find themselves sitting in classrooms in which they have been teaching for much of the day. Take into account the impact of location on members. Since one of the disadvantages of group consultation is attendance problems, the consultant may need to deal with this issue of location. Attendance is a problem throughout the process, but it is worst in the initial stages of consultation. Attendance has an impact on the development of cohesion and productivity in the group. So problems are best addressed by preventing their beginning with careful planning, scheduling, selection of members, and effective group skills on the part of the leader (Brown, Wyne, Blackburn, and Powell, 1979).

Problem resolution is a key part of the group leader's role. When the leader is able to use the multiple problem-solving potential offered by a group of people, the group approach becomes advantageous to problem resolution (Shaw, 1976). The leader can encourage comments from certain group members, or use guided statements, or direct suggestions toward problem solving. This is done within the context of creative problem solving activity. Dinkmeyer (1971) suggests that group dynamics which add to this process include a heterogeneous group, such as a mix of variously experienced teachers—experienced, inexperienced, older, younger, and with different orientations to educational approaches. However, it usually works best to incorporate members who are able to share some similar interests. Encouraging group involvement reduces dependency on the leader. The group leader has as a goal the independence of the members. Nelson and Shefron (1985) describe the primary goal of consultation to be helping consultees become more efficient, effective, independent, and resourceful in their abilities to solve the problems they face. These guidelines lend themselves well to a collaborative model. The goal of group members' independence will necessarily shape the role of the leader. The group leader will not always be available to the consultees in the future and encourages them toward independence.

The group leader's role is developed in response to the group members' needs and presents skills. The consultation group leader initiates a collaborative role with the consultees. One way of developing such a collaborative relationship is to minimize differences in status, or the power hierarchy, so that consultees and consultant can function as collaborators in the problem-solving venture. If the consultant does not have an evaluative function, it is important to make this clear, since the consultant who is not evaluating the consultees' work is in a better position to build this type of collaborative relationship. If the consultant has accepted the position of evaluator within the institution, the consultant should know what this means to his/her role and describe it to the consultees. This factor cannot be ignored by either party; however, it should be handled so that the relationship is not impeded.

Establishing the role of collaborator with consultees is an approach which can facilitate the group process. Caplan (1970) describes a technique used by consultants to develop the collaborator role called "one-downmanship," in which the consultant answers the consultee by deferring back to the consultee. In this way of communicating the consultant and consultee are equals. Another approach, using anecdotes, is described by Berlin (1967). The consultant uses anecdotes which illustrate difficult experiences the consultant has had. This should make the consultee feel at ease about any feelings of unsureness or anxiety. It should be noted, however, that as helpful as these techniques may be, they can be overused. The consultant then may appear to have nothing to offer the consultee, in which case the collaborative relationship can hardly help.

Assisting consultees to form realistic expectations for the group consultation experience is an important aspect of the leader's role. Because there are many members, many expectations will exist. This can become overwhelming when these expectations are not revealed and reality-tested. Selzer (1981) describes the problem of hidden agendas in the case conference format. Hidden agendas are wishes or needs often played out in relation to the consultant. Staff members may want the consultant to act in certain ways, such as to align with a subgroup, or sanction a particular position, or confront certain members whom others are too afraid to confront. Selzer warns that the consultant must trust reactions within the group, which will yield important information about the staff. The consultant may ignore this information out of a wish to remain objective and removed. Yet often these are signs of the dynamics which are going on in the agency, between staff, and possibly clients. Recognizing this enables the consultant to assist the staff in identifying the dynamics and responding in new ways. Consultants need to help consultees to form realistic expectations of the group process and of the leader. It is not uncommon for members to wish the leader would offer direct solutions to a problem. They may hope for a diagnosis and prescription to fix the problem. Or they may wish the consultant would take the responsibility for the cure away from them. Consultees with these kinds of expectations, or with hidden agendas, frequently leave the group experience early unless their expectations are clarified and sometimes challenged. The consultant needs to spend time assisting consultees in describing their expectations. The consultant can then describe the realistic outcomes for the consultation group. The rest is process. The consultant models persistence in resolving problems and presents clear communication about outcomes.

Group consultees need to be assisted in forming clear expectations and they are invited into a collaborative relationship. These factors are part of a healthy contract between the group leader and the members of the consultee group. The leader is wise to lead in a relatively group-centered fashion. Consultees expect that they will be involved in a decision or in collaborative problem solving. This involves delegating certain tasks, consulting group members about problem diagnoses as well as problem solutions. It may also mean allowing the group to have decision-making functions. This is particularly useful when the consultant is with the group long enough to teach skills that can be used on a regular basis after the consultant is no longer present.

GROUP CONSULTATION DYNAMICS

The dynamics of group consultation closely resemble those of group counseling. A group consultant needs to have experience leading groups as well as an understanding of the consultation process. Group dynamics may present issues to the leader of a consultation group. An understanding of these concerns is important. Issues which can assist in elaborating the group consultation process are group cohesion, communication, and resistance. The typical stages of group consultation, how one selects the right group consultation approach, and ethical issues will also be addressed.

Group Cohesion

Group cohesion means a feeling is shared by the group members that each individual has a place in it (Hansen, Warner, and Smith, 1980). A sense of oneness of purpose is developed, and it is this purpose which binds the members together. The members have a feeling of being part of something special. This, as well as individual importance felt by members, holds the group together as a unit. Consequently, a cohesive group is a stable and productive group that can be quite task or goal oriented (Gazda, 1984).

The group consultation leader would do well to reinforce member involvement and facilitate group cohesiveness. One way to do this is to assist members in identifying with the purpose of the group. The leader can show members how they relate to the topics being discussed. This is done by tying people together and by connecting people in various ways to the issue at hand. For example, two members of a teacher consultation group discuss their frustrations in dealing with parents. The group leader recognizes each contribution and links them together in a common way, showing a shared feeling of frustration. Frustration is expressed openly and developed so others can add their own similar feelings. Support is provided for each person who has spoken and shared their feelings on a particular issue. This recognition reinforces their place in the group and models acceptance of participation. It is quite helpful for quiet members who are more reluctant in group activity. This type of connecting behavior on the part of the group leader facilitates overall group cohesion.

Cohesion may be enhanced by openly discussing differing points of view in the group. One cannot expect all members to agree or understand in the same way. Cohesion should not be confused with agreement or even friendship. However, when discord or disharmony exists, the cohesive group can move through this with the help of the leader. The leader is wise to express the differing concerns fairly and objectively, offering credence to both. It is helpful to show appreciation for the insight of a member with statements such as, "That's a good point you have raised." The member is affirmed for contributing to the overall direction of the group. Or the leader can acknowledge a differing position by saying, "That is another way of looking at the same issue." The leader should state that all members come with their own set of experiences which shape how things are viewed, and describe the benefit of learning from each other. The group leader can then proceed by drawing the focus of the group back to the overall goal. When integration of differing views is pursued in conjunction with the group's overall purpose and with respect for the members, behavior is modeled by the leader which can result in openness, acceptance, and future problem resolution.

Communication

It may seem obvious that communication is a significant part of group dynamics. Yet, the dynamics of the group consultation process depend on communication. Communication is an issue in terms of presenting the problem; handling the problem; and dealing with the member who presents the issue.

The consultee may need assistance in describing the problem. The issue could be so heavy with personal feelings that communication is impeded and, consequently, the group has difficulty understanding the meaning of the problem to the consultee. The leader and group members need to ask questions to help clarify the description of the problem. The consultee learns that his or her presentation was not clear and is perhaps ambiguous. Through this experience of clarification everyone can learn that data from a variety of sources must be put together along with the experiential data to form a clearer picture of the etiology of the problem. Sources the consultee can draw on to develop the fuller picture may include, in a school setting, other school personnel with whom the client has interacted, the student's family life as reported by family or others, or, in the case of a youth counselor in a probation setting, other staff may have input/experiences, or teachers may contribute behavior descriptions from school, or the family may describe home visits. Such data, gathered and presented along with the consultee's experiential data, form a clearer and less ambiguous picture. They also provide a more objective presentation to which the group can respond.

The consultant must be sensitive to the consultee's inner experience in presenting the case. All communication the consultant offers should be attuned to any possible conflicts the consultee may feel, the consultee's need to protect self-esteem, the need to avoid anxiety, the need to control his/her environment, or even the need to reject any level of dependency. McDaniel, Weber, and Wynne (1986) refer to avoiding "de-skilling the consultee" and encourage the consultant to recognize feelings of inadequacy in the consultee. The consultant must provide the needed expertise while supporting the strengths of the system and the people within it. This task needs to be accomplished without increasing any feelings of inadequacy that might have motivated the consultation request. The consultant can address any of these inner feelings in subtle ways by simply remaining calm, accepting the feelings expressed, and interacting with the consultee as a colleague. The consultant can help the consultee become more comfortable with the process of exploring and be more objective in dealing with the important aspects of the case. Anxiety lessens and the consultee is able to view the positive aspects of his/her contribution to the client and consider what else may be done to assist the client. A leader's awareness of non-verbal communication is useful. All individuals communicate simultaneously in this way, even if only one member is talking at a time. Scanning becomes more helpful than maintaining eye contact with one person. Cues of support, disagreement, anxiety, eagerness, and other aspects of involvement can be determined by the leader.

Consultation in a group is a more complex and, in many ways, a more demanding experience for the consultees. Each member is usually encouraged to participate in all consultees' cases. A community effort is experienced, all members contributing and helping. The individual member cannot be only self-focused. At the same time, the group member can gain from each experience presented. Consequently, the learning is greater. Consultees are able to confront a number of issues. For example, a youth counselor may look at: substance abuse; family dynamics; behavioral change; developmental stages of youth; the impact of schools, home, church, and other institutions on youth; and personal dynamics one must be aware of in working with youth. The consultee learns not from just one case review but from many others presented within the group setting. In addition, the consultee learns many more communication behaviors by participating in a group consultation. When a consultee is alone in consultation, the consultee has the undivided attention of the consultant; the issue of group dynamics does not exist. The helping process in a group setting flows not only between the consultant and the consultee, but also among the group members themselves (Drapela, 1983). In a group setting, there are issues about who speaks to whom; whether it is appropriate to say something to the presenting consultee; whether it is okay to offer suggestions from one's own experience; and how opinions from others are accepted. The group leader invites questions, opinions, and suggestions or comments. The consultant becomes a model of nonjudgmental analysis which the group consultees use to learn to help each other. Consultees will learn which comments tend to facilitate the problem-solving journey. Eventually, it becomes easier for individuals to contribute and for the group to develop a sense of cohesiveness and cooperation.

Resistance

Resistance often comes from a reluctance to be involved in the group process and/or to address personal issues. Group rules can help protect the rights of individual members and promote a nonthreatening, creative group climate. The rules offer an assurance to group members that their individuality and personal freedom will be respected as long as they are willing to respect the rights of others. The concept of group rules can be positively oriented in this way and seen as protection rather than an intrusion. Resistance is best dealt with in an atmosphere where all members are beginning to trust. Individuals within the group will connect with the group norm of speaking and responding openly. They will become more closely identified with the purpose of the group. Resistance within individuals can often be reduced by creating a safe, trusting environment.

The problem of resistance can be more than individual. It may exist outside of the group and be system-centered. There are many institutions which promote group response and heavily influence the behavior of the members (Brown, Wyne, Blackburn, and Powell, 1979). It is reasonable to assume that member participation in consultation will be influenced by the group. Consultants need to deal with individual members, yet, at the same time, realize the impact on the group. Resistance must be considered both an individual and a group phenomenon.

Berlin (1979) describes the awareness mental health consultants need in order to resolve institutions' resistance to change. Institutions frequently employ consultants to help solve problems, yet, when this involves change, there are mechanisms to resist or stop the change. Some common methods of institutional resistance include: creating inertia, made up of anxiety about change, which results in no action; delays and vagueness about the plan which result in people giving up on the plan of action; the assignment of committees to study the changes, often selected without leadership or with people not in favor of the change which results in inaction; well-developed plans are placed in the hands of inept administrators or those committed to the status quo, which results in a dead end for the plan; or administrators ensure that splinter groups exist which results in no unified approach to the action. Berlin also warns that organizations may use consultation to avoid change. One of the most confusing and effective ways of making sure that change does not occur is for an expert to be hired to defend against change. It is essential that the consultant understand the dynamics of the institution by obtaining a thorough knowledge of the institution, its history, and its problems. The consultant should also listen to "front-line" workers. These approaches will assist in identifying any resistance and will eventually help in addressing it.

STAGES OF GROUP CONSULTATION

The stages of group consulting generally follow those of group counseling. We can identify the stages as entry, diagnosis and intervention, and termination. These stages will be described briefly within the context of a group consultation case.

Entry

The entry stage in group consulting consists of the initial contact with the agency or institution. This stage is critical developmentally since the consultation contract is created during this stage. The initial organization and planning work takes place now. The role of consultant is established and, consequently, also that of the consultee(s).

A mental health consultant was invited into a consultation with the faculty and staff of a Native American elementary school. The consultant had an education background as well as some knowledge of the culture of the Native American people. The consultant was known to the staff and faculty from previous parent education training programs and teacher consultations. The invitation was initiated by the principal, who was concerned about staff and faculty relations. His specific concern was in the area of communication.

The consultant met with the principal and developed a general contract for eight weeks of one-hour sessions once each week. It was agreed the principal would participate since he recognized he was part of the communication system. The contract was written with a general purpose of improving the communication dynamics of the staff. It was the intention of the consultant to expand the specifics when meeting the first time with the group, rather than determining the direction without their input.

The teachers of the six grade levels, the librarian, the secretarial staff, the teacher assistant, resource teaching staff, and the principal met together in the consultation sessions. The first meeting was part of entry; it was used to more specifically develop the contract. The members of the group were asked to describe their concerns, problems, and worries about staff relations and communication. Many examples of problem situations were referred to without any judging or diagnosis offered. The consultant attempted to establish a role of collaborator with the staff.

Diagnosis and Intervention

Diagnosis in group consulting needs to be an ongoing process. It begins with the entry stage and continues through termination. All data become part of the way of understanding the population, the problem, and addressing the issues. The purpose of intervention in this type of consultation is to enter into a human system of relationships with the goal of making a helpful difference (Kurpius, 1985). If done properly, interventions can transform systems. Influence can be initiated in the proper places, deficits can be altered for the promotion of assets, and a climate for creative problem solving is developed.

In the case of the staff consultation group, there was a necessary overlap of entry, diagnosis, and intervention. The consultant needed to gather more information for a clear contract and to confirm the approach of an eight-week program in the first session. This, however, was the first week of an intervention program. This is quite appropriate when the consultant has a base of understanding about the system and the consultees and is familiar with the specific institution. It is also appropriate when using the process model. Selecting the proper intervention must be preceded by understanding the problem context.

The consultant wants to develop a diagnosis which assesses the system variables, such as multicultural differences, ownership of the problem, and determining the readiness of consultees. The consultant working with the staff and faculty of the Native American elementary school needed to recognize the system variables. The principal and all teaching staff, with the exception of the teaching assistant, were white. All other staff, which embodied the support staff, were Native American. The school was located on the reservation where only Native American students attended. It was therefore necessary that the consultant address the cultural variables that existed and which likely created some tension in communication and staff development.

The diagnosis was focused on the cultural differences of the staff and the faculty as well as the professional distinction which existed in the different roles of the two groups. The intervention was established around these differences so as to provide opportunity to minimize the differences and increase clear communication. The purpose of this intervention was to increase communication and interaction between work groups, to reduce dysfunctional competition, and to replace independent views with an awareness of the necessity for interdependent action.

The intervention consisted of the eight weekly sessions focusing on cultural differences and communication patterns within the system. Since cultural difference was one of the main issues, such differences were the initial focus of the consultation. The other issue was that of the differing roles within the elementary school, with the White population represented in the professional positions and the Native Americans represented as support staff. To begin with, the consultant established time for all participants to present background information on their individual cultures. This type of sharing was done casually, informally, and within a confidential setting. The consultant intentionally modeled the role of collaborator. This role was going to be very instrumental in the future developing roles of all consultees. The group proceeded with a great deal of sharing, which was educational for everyone but especially for the teaching faculty. They had not had, or taken, the opportunity to understand the Native American culture from an objective point of view. Responses to the material were encouraged. The reactions to some of the material, especially of white oppression of Native Americans, was strained. The atmosphere was at times tense. Trust was not always possible. All these experiences needed to be analyzed in the context of the school system.

During the course of the eight weeks, the consultant began tying together patterns of historical misinformation and misinterpretation, lack of trust, subtle and not-so-subtle oppression of Native Americans by whites, and the ignorance of the oppressors. These patterns were not evident in the daily actions and communication of the school. This type of background, however, fed into a long history of perceptions on the part of both groups. This was addressed in an atmosphere characterized by a high degree of caring, respect, and common concern. Trust was building within this environment. The differences were not eliminated, but they were beginning to diminish.

Since the teaching staff was white and the support staff was Native American, the issue of role differences was also addressed. One way was to begin to understand how this was the case. Many of the staff knew that Native Americans were sought by this particular principal for teaching positions. This had not proved fruitful. Yet, the staff knew there was a genuine desire to hire Native Americans as teachers. It was a continual concern being addressed at the school. As far as the support staff was concerned, only Native Americans were permitted to work in these positions. All agreed it was very helpful to the white teachers to have the resources of these individuals; they were able to describe some of the Native American ways to the teachers. The consultant taught communication skills to all staff using structured activities and then applied these skills to the communication of the system. The issue of role difference was addressed in part, along with cultural differences. Communication patterns were assessed and suggestions were made for changes. During the eight weeks, the consultant had the opportunity to assign communication tasks to the staff. They tried these new models out and returned to the group to discuss their efforts. Once the major issues of cultural difference were discussed and trust began to build, the communication patterns were taught quite easily. People were much more willing to approach others; moving across one another's boundaries, into territory that was now not so frightening. This process was most often positively received and at times welcomed.

Termination

Termination is better seen as part of the consultation process rather than a stage. When viewed as a stage, we often do not consider termination until we are about to exit the door of the program. This is a mistake. Termination should be on the mind of the consultant very early in the process. Termination is part of the diagnosis. The consultant will ask questions about the dependence of the group, about the readiness of the group, about the developing outcomes of the goals, and many more questions which will assist the consultant in determining how termination will be effected.

Termination in the Native American school began when behavior (and attitude) change began to develop in the group. When the maintenance of these behaviors was evident, termination was timely. It is at this stage that we see group autonomy begin to develop. The group needs the consultant less and less. The consultant is no longer the center of the communication focus. All members share the responsibility of and for communication. The members are able to use one another as resource people and to facilitate problem solving. The consultant began to hear of frequent occasions during the week when many issues formerly addressed only in the group were being discussed in the staff lunch room, in the secretary's office, and after hours in the classrooms and halls. Termination is a time to celebrate behavior change and to recognize that the consultant is no longer needed.

All stages are important in the group consultation process. Each deserves the consultant's full attention and concern. It is also important to note that all stages evolve into each other. There is seldom a clear distinction between them; this is the characteristic of group process. The consultant should be cautious not to get stuck on any one stage (Russ, 1978). This may happen when one member is not progressing at the rate of the others. The consultant may be reluctant to move on, fearing leaving a member behind. However, the consultant needs to trust the function of the group. The group will often have more power over a reluctant member than the leader. The group as a whole needs to address this type of issue. Sometimes the consultant will get stuck at one particular stage she or he is feeling pretty good about where the group is; or, more critically, she or he is unwilling to take the next move because it may require confrontation. In these cases it remains important for the consultant to remember that the goal of consultation is for the consultant not to be needed anymore. Good feelings come from the development of independent consultees who have gained important behaviors and understandings from the experience of the consultation.

ISSUES

The selection of group consultation over individual consultation must be made using a number of considerations. In some circumstances the areas to consider become advantages; in others there are disadvantages for a particular approach. The consultant has several determinations to make, such as consultant skills, consultee needs, and time available.

Consultant skills should determine the model used. If a consultant is inadequate in group work, the individual consultation model is better suited. Productive group work rests heavily on group leader skills. The trained group leader does not use group consultation exclusively but recognizes particular needs of individuals who will not benefit from the group approach and who may very well impede the group process.

Consultee needs and the goal of the consultation can be used to guide the choice of group consultation. When the consultee is presenting a case, for example, with confidential material, it may be advised to work with this person on an individual basis rather than in a group. This approach will reduce the problems associated with confidentiality regarding other group members. It will also eliminate the possibility that group members cannot relate to the material presented in a delicate case. The group approach, however, is best used when all group members can identify with the concerns presented and topics discussed. In fact, the group process extends the benefits of consultation.

Group work is mutually shared with a collaborative approach. It is well suited for situations where topics are being presented for the education and training of the consultees. Communication skills and behavior change can be presented to parents, conflict management and crisis intervention can be presented to youth-home employees, and family dynamics and domestic disputes can be presented to police officers. In each, the group has similar goals and works with the same population so that the group process can be moved in a common direction. The group's members have the opportunity to learn from one another and "process" the material presented. Group work is also well suited for case review. Case work can be done in conjunction with the presentation of topical information or alone as a consultation program. Many groups of professionals gain from the opportunity to "run" a case with a consultant. Tomlinson (1981) describes handling multiple cases in schools when time is limited. A consultant can meet with a small group of teachers responsible for children with similar behavior problems. In this approach, more time can be allowed to describe the general analysis and approach to the type of problem in question. This increases the likelihood that the teachers may generalize the approach to similar problems. The group approach also provides an opportunity for teachers to assist each other in developing ways of implementing certain procedures. Group work is mutually shared whereas the individual approach may be better suited for unique cases, or cases with highly personal information.

The group approach is an excellent model when working within a system and addressing the issues, problems, and even resistance within the institution (Gadlin, 1985; Nelson and Shefron, 1985; Berlin, 1979; and Sbordone and Sterman, 1983). The group approach permits educative counterefforts which may be more effective in changing the system on a broader scale than in working with an individual or even a series of individuals. The group process may be more empowering for those employees who have lost any sense of control in their work. It may be used to deal with the group as a system within a system. The group as a system can adjust and alter behavior which will impact the overall system. Understanding the institution as a system and then using the group process to approach the issues of the system means the consultant will direct attention to the interactions between people and between hierarchy levels. This prevents exclusive concentration on the inadequacies of one part of the system (Gadlin, 1985). The system is viewed as a total entity with the working group a part of it. When the consultant wishes to address concerns systemic in nature, one approach is to deal with the consultation within a group setting. The group setting allows some of the aspects of the system to become apparent and be addressed.

Group consultation is difficult to organize in a situation of crisis. It is highly unlikely a group can meet quickly to deal with the crises that may arise for its members. Consequently, it is recommended that crises be handled on an individual basis (Brown, Wyne, Blackburn, and Powell, 1979). The exception are settings where the staff are organized to respond to crises in a group or team approach. For example, the staff at a mental health center may already be organized into teams that process and approach cases together. In the event of a crisis, the team, used to working together and accustomed to handling crises, can quickly meet to confront a particular circumstance that may come up. There are advantages to groups facing crises together. One is when the leader is unavailable. When the person who normally conducts the approach to crisis is not accessible, a member may be able to contact other members and organize a helpful approach based on what the group has learned from past experience with the group leader. This works well, especially when the group has developed a cohesive, trusting, and supportive environment.

Group consultation lends itself to a variety of programs. It is useful in education programs such as parent education, or case review programs where case conferencing or supervision sessions with counselors are conducted. The group consultation process as a collaborative approach makes use of the exchange of ideas and support between members. It has the potential for creative problem resolution. Group experiences are particularly appropriate when consultants want to generate communication or improve the communication process. Dialogue among staff in a system where dialogue has not been especially productive is a good use of the group consultation approach. This type of process makes use of the systems approach and group relations (Kaslow, 1986; Fisher, 1986).

The Ethics of Confidentiality

Since consultants have no particular set of rules that govern their behavior apart from those in effect for their other professional functions (Conoley and Conoley, 1982), they find themselves facing complex situations without guidelines. One of the most likely circumstances a consultant will experience is the dilemma of confidentiality. It is a conflict that should be expected. The consultant is best prepared for issues of confidentiality by understanding his/her own values of human behavior and by knowing the ethical and legal responsibilities of the field of consultation, and in terms of the agency and client population. Objectivity will assist the consultant in this discerning; discernment is an important aspect of employing professional behavior regarding confidentiality. The consultant needs to avoid the cheap thrill of being told "confidential information." All helping relationships require a degree of confidentiality (Drapela, 1983), all helping relationships require a professional response to the issue of confidentiality.

A responsible consultant will address the inevitable issue of confidentiality at the beginning of the consultation relationship. The consultant's commitment to confidentiality should be mentioned during the entry process (Conoley and Conoley, 1982). The consultant may have ideas about confidentiality based on past experiences. However, each group situation can be different enough to require variations in confidential agreements. Brown, Wyne, Blackburn, and Powell (1979) suggest the norm of confidentiality should be set on a group-to-group basis, with members determining whether material will be kept in confidence. Members need to observe the degree of confidentiality agreed on by the group (Drapela, 1983). The agreed-upon rules of confidentiality will remain a continuing concern for all involved. All parties in the consultation process are professionals and should be prepared to accept responsibility for confidentiality. The consultant can lead this behavior by assisting in definition and by modeling. The maintenance of the confidentiality agreement is essential to developing and encouraging trust in the total experience.

Certain situations will require that information formerly identified as confidential be shared outside the group. The issue of client welfare must be the guideline in this event. When confidentialities need to be broken, all parties should be informed. The consultant may also be placed in a situation where someone in the institution but outside the group asks for information considered by the consultant to be confidential. For example, a school consultant may be approached by an administrator for information about a teacher in the group. It is wise for the consultant to refer to the contract developed at the entry stage. If the contract prohibits sharing of this kind of material and there is no emergency presented by the administrator, the consultant proceeds according to the contract. Usually this means that any information shared formally or otherwise must be either already public or offered only after permission is given by the teacher. Public information includes the work a teacher does which can be observed by others, such as hall behavior, class response to a new experience, or the integration of a handicapped child into the classroom. Even positive statements about a teacher should not be shared unless permission is given. It should never be assumed the consultant will select information which will not hurt the teacher. For example, when a statement of praise for one teacher is shared among the staff, the impact may be that of vicious competition. It is always important to remember the teacher is part of a total system, and the theory of systems tells us that the behavior change of one person will impact on the others. We need to appreciate the fact that at times this impact may be negative.

The consultant would do well to assume much of the responsibility for the definition of confidentiality in group consultation. However, it is impossible to monitor all members' behavior regarding the agreement. Feldman (1979) reminds us that consultation is a collaborative process and we need to educate consultees to assume the responsibilities that accompany this role. Consultants and consultees alike need to recognize that the consultation process involves some degree of power to make decisions and carry out choices but, in addition, involves the accompanying responsibility. The consultant can model, encourage professional behavior, and deal openly with the issue. Yet confidentiality will remain a potential problem, and become a greater problem the larger the number of people. Recognizing this may result in additional caution. In the event the consultant or anyone else is involved in a breach of confidence made unknowingly, the person(s) should go immediately to the injured party and explain the circumstances. Recognition of human frailty does no one harm and likely will result in more caution in the future as well as a level of respect for the honesty shared. Valuing confidentiality is a clear example of a person's commitment to relationships developed between people.

Multicultural Concerns

Ethnic differences as applied to the consultation process have not received much attention in research (Mannino, MacLennan, and Shore, 1975). In studies directly relevant to Blacks, for example, Gibbs (1980) notes most research deals with lower-class Blacks and inner-city ghetto communities, limiting the applicability to other groups. She adds, however, that some shared traits and patterns exist. Gibbs developed a model of interpersonal orientation to consulting based on a synthesis of research findings. She identified stages of consultation with Blacks and themes which reflect an interpersonal orientation of black consultees to the consultation relationship. Gibbs suggests a more interpersonal orientation of Black consultees in contrast with the instrumental orientation of white consultees. This emphasizes the need to use the interpersonal mode with Black consultees. For example, the consultant's ability to use nontechnical language and communicate to members at all levels of the system is a positive factor in the early stage for Blacks. At this stage of appraisal and assessment the consultant may be able to equalize the differences between consultant and consultee(s). This can also be true at the stage of involvement when the consultee is evaluating the consultant's degree of identification with his/her ethnic background. An example of this is a group consultation conducted by white mental health consultants in a mental health project with predominantly black, inner-city youth workers. The task was to train the youth workers in interpersonal skills, crisis intervention responses, communication skills, and problem-solving skills. The trainees were to apply these skills in their work with inner-city youth, primarily in playground settings. The consultants were well prepared for the technical and instrumental orientation with the consultees. However, they were not adequately prepared for the process orientation of this population and the impact on their view of their roles. Racial and cultural issues influenced the relationships with the consultants and impacted the learning process. Use of nontechnical language was necessary to bridge a teaching/learning relationship. It was important for the consultants to relate as people rather than as authorities with expertise. It was important to communicate to all levels of the consultee system. In an attempt to equalize differences a sports activity was planned in which the youth were bound to excel. This provided a common experience between the two groups, an experience to which the teaching material could be applied. Most importantly, it permitted a beginning for the needed interpersonal orientation with this population. The implication of Gibb's model is that the interpersonal competence of the consultant must initially be evaluated before instrumental competence is demonstrated. The equalization of differences between consultant(s) and consultee(s) must be considered an important part of the entry stage in consultation, especially where multicultural differences exist.

Directions for Research

Research on individual psychotherapy has grown; however, research on the processes and outcome of consultation has fallen behind (Wynne, McDaniel, and Weber, 1986). The focus of research has been on the characteristics of consultation, with little attention on the study of goals and outcomes. It seems the practice of consultation has expanded beyond the theoretical foundations for consultation. The early work does not answer all the questions. Gallessich (1985) suggests research priorities be shifted to address basic questions regarding the nature of consultation by constructing a meta-theory. Here general characteristics of the different consultation approaches are identified then related to a higher-order conceptualization. This would unify similarities among approaches. Another way is to identify the differences so as to lead to newer, more cogent theories.

Kellogg (1984) conducted research studying the establishment of successful consulting relationships within groups. She found the problem areas of consulting relationships were areas where both consultee and consultant have some control. Both participants are called to take initiatives to improve the quality of this relationship. The three areas which contribute to it are: the matching process, the clear contract, and communication. First, in the matching process the consultant may recognize the need for a choice not to work with someone. Should the choice be made to work with a consultee, however, the establishment of a mutual relationship is very important to the consultation relationship. Second, a clear contract is necessary. Kellogg suggests the contract be not only clear but limited for specificity. In addition, it should be a contract of genuine interest to the consultee. The third area regards clear communication. This research may contribute to future exploration in the direction of the collaborative relationship between consultants and consultees.

The procedural approach in consultation was examined by Hugo Prein (1984) in a research study comparing it and its characteristic process-orientation with third-party confrontation and mediation. The procedural approach is the most successful because it has stronger implications in consultation and has broader applications than either confrontation or mediation. Important qualities in the procedural approach include: the mutual relationship, creating and realizing solutions, and the process-oriented style with emphasis on identifying problems, decision making, and problem solving. These mutual-relationship qualities could be assessed in terms of the collaborative relationship described by Kellogg.

Swierczek (1980) researched the nature of collaborative intervention in organizational change. The outcome of this study suggests there may not be a strong relationship between collaboration and success. There may be little association between collaborative problem definition, collaborative solution, and effectiveness. This does not mean there is no relationship between collaborative intervention and successful organizational change. Yet, questions are created by this research which need to be examined. We can say collaboration is important in accomplishing change, but it is only part of the systematic and well-designed strategy for intervention in consultation.

If we agree that consultation is based on role and relationship rules

(Gallessich, 1985), then we need to address the research already done and look toward continued research in this area. The relationship is voluntary and collaborative. Both consultant and consultee retain responsibility and authority for actions (Gallessich, 1985). We would be wise to promote further research in this area. In addition, we need to look at the impact of multicultural concerns.

Many have addressed the connection between the multicultural background of the consultant and consultee(s) (Gallessich, 1985; Gibbs, 1985; and Inouye and Pedersen, 1985). Directions for consultation research need to take into consideration multicultural populations. Inouye and Pedersen (1985) reviewed the cultural and ethnic content of APA convention programs over a six-year period. They found little time (5.6 percent) was devoted to general cultural processes or national, racial, or ethnic groups. The amount of time did not increase over the years reviewed in spite of the stated policy in support of cultural awareness. There appears to be a discrepancy between professed goals and reality of concern. Cultural variables do have a bearing on the ethicality of our endeavors. Effects of culture are suited for methodological exploration (Inouye and Pedersen, 1985). Further research is needed with all consultation populations. Studies need to pair consultants and consultees in varying ways. Gibbs (1980) suggests using interracial teams of consultants to deliver services to interracial consultee staffs. In these kinds of studies, it becomes essential to also investigate the impact of sex, status, power, and age.

The brevity of most consultative relationships creates practical problems for research design (Wynne, McDaniel, and Weber, 1986). Gathering background information necessary for the research may take as much time as the actual consultation. Yet, this background data could be seen as helpful and useful to the consultant in many aspects of the consultation process. It is not wasted time. This is especially true for consultation which leads to therapeutic decisions. The additional research conducted prior to consultation for the purposes of methodological exploration, could be useful in the therapy outcome.

It is desirable to research the models of consultation with families and groups. Research has fallen behind the general practice of consultation. Studies such as consulting outcome and cost-effectiveness should be carried out. It is also desirable to research the role of consultant. With so much focus on the consultant as collaborator, we need to identify the dynamics of this role within hierarchical institutions and within a variety of systems. In addition, we need to recognize culture within the consultation process. At the international level, in an atmosphere of increasing interdependency among nations, a greater knowledge of other nationalities is essential. At the national level, it is necessary for consultants to address multicultural variables while striving toward an improved understanding of our diverse population (Inouye and Pedersen, 1985). The lack of addressing the differences among the various populations limits productivity and outcome but, what is worse, it shows a narrowness and limited perspective which we cannot afford in our world today.

SUMMARY

Consultation is a vehicle for bringing needed knowledge and services to modern work organizations (Gallessich, 1985). Consultants may approach groups and organizations through hierarchy structures and may address leadership, quality of work, skills needed for effecting change, interpersonal relationships, and so forth. The consultant's time frame may be a factor in the decision to use group consultation. In the long term, the group approach is cost-effective. In the short term, it meets the needs of more consultees and ultimately impacts more clients. However, planning and organizing are more complicated and time-consuming for group consultation than for individual consultation. Individual consultation may be the better approach when a consultee shows a need somewhat isolated from those of colleagues and quick response is an issue. On the other hand, if there is enough time to organize a program which responds to the needs of several people, the effort to plan a group consultation would be worthwhile. Generally, the decision to use a group approach is the consultant's. The decision should be made giving consideration to the skills of the consultant, the time constraints and, always and uppermost, the needs of the consultee(s).

REFERENCES

BERLIN, I. (1979). Resistance to mental health consultation directed at change in public institutions. *Community Mental Health Journal*, 15 (2), 119–128.

BERLIN, I. (1967). Preventive aspects of mental health consultation to schools. *Mental Hygiene*, 51, 340.

BROWN, D., WYNE, M., BLACKBURN, J., and POWELL, W. (1979). *Consultation: Strategy for improving education*. Boston: Allyn and Bacon.

CAPLAN, G. (1970). *The theory and practice of mental health consultation*. New York: Basic Books.

CONOLEY, J., and CONOLEY, C. (1982). The effects of two conditions of client-centered consultation on student teacher problem descriptions and remedial plans. *Journal of School Psychology*, 20 (4), 323–328.

DINKMEYER, D. (1971). The "C" group: Integrating knowledge and experience to change behavior, an adlerian approach to consultation. *The Counseling Psychologist*, 3 (1), 63–72.

DRAPELA, V. (1983). *The counselor as consultant and supervisor*. Springfield, IL: Charles C. Thomas.

FELDMAN, R. (1979). Collaborative consultation: A process for joint professional–consumer development of primary prevention programs. *Journal of Community Psychology*, 7, 118–128.

GADLIN, W. (1985). Psychiatric consultation to the medical ward: A group analytic and general systems theory point of view. *International Journal, Group Psychotherapy*, 35 (2), 263–277.

GALLESSICH, J. (1985). Toward a meta-theory of consultation. *The Counseling Psychologist*, 13 (3), 336–354.

GAZDA, G. (1984). *Group counseling: A developmental approach.* Boston: Allyn and Bacon.

GIBBS, J. (1985). Can we continue to be color-blind and class-bound? *The Counseling Psychologist*, 13 (3), 426–435.

GIBBS, J. (1980). The interpersonal orientation in mental health consultation: Toward a model of ethic variations in consultation. *Journal of Community Psychology*, 8, 195–207.

HANSON, J., WARNER, R., and SMITH, E. (1980). *Group counseling.* Chicago: Rand McNally Publishing Co.

INOUYE, K., and PEDERSEN, P. (1985). Cultural and ethnic content of the 1977 to 1982 American Psychological Association convention programs. *The Counseling Psychologist*, 13 (4), 639–648.

KASLOW, F. (1986). Consultation with the military: A complex role. In L. Wynne, S. McDaniel, and T. Weber (eds.), *Systems consultation: A new perspective for family therapy*, (383–397). New York: The Guilford Press.

KELLOGG, D. (1984). Contrasting successful and unsuccessful organizational development consultation relationships. *Group and Organizational Studies*, 9 (2), 151–188.

KURPIUS, D. (1985). Consultation interventions: Successes, failures and proposals. *The Counseling Psychologist*, 13 (3), 368–389.

MANNINO, F., MACLENNAN, B., and SHORE, M. (1975). *The practice of mental health consultation.* Washington, DC: U.S. Government Printing Office.

MCDANIEL, S., WEBER, T., and WYNNE, L. (1986). Consultants at the crossroads: Problems and controversies in systems consultation. In L. Wynne, S. McDaniel, and T. Weber (eds.), *Systems consultation: A new perspective for family therapy* (449–462). New York: The Guilford Press.

NELSON, R., and SHEFRON, R. (1985). Choice awareness in consultation. *Counselor Education and Supervision*, 24 (3), 298–306.

PREIN, H. (1984). A contingency approach for conflict intervention. *Group and Organizational Studies*, 9 (1), 81–102.

RUSS, S. (1978). Group consultation: Key variables that effect change. *Professional Psychology*, February, 145–152.

SBORDONE, R., and STERMAN, L. (1983). The psychologist as a consultant in a nursing home: Effect on staff morale and turnover. *Professional Psychology: Research and Practice*, 14 (2), 240–250.

SELZER, M. (1981). The role of the consultant in the case conference: Some neglected aspects. *Psychiatry*, 44, February, 60–68.

SHAW, M., (1976). *Group dynamics: The psychology of small group behavior*, 2nd ed. New York: McGraw Hill.

SWIERCZEK, F. (1980). Collaborative intervention and participation in organizational change. *Group and Organizational Studies*, 5 (4), 438–452.

Tomlinson, J. (1981). Implementing behavior modification programs with limited consultation time. In M. Curtis, and J. Zins, *The theory and practice of school consultation*. Springfield, IL: Charles C. Thomas.

Wynne, L., McDaniel, S., and Weber, T. (1986). Future directions for systems consultation. In L. Wynne, S. McDaniel, and T. Weber (eds.), *Systems consultation: A new perspective for family therapy* (463–475). New York: The Guilford Press.

CHAPTER SEVEN
CONSULTATION WITH FAMILIES

This chapter will address family consultation based on the systems theory. Family consultation is a brief and powerful encounter between the parties involved. It adds insight for the professionals and dimension to their practice. New skills, knowledge, and understandings are available to the consultee–therapist through consultation. The family consultation interchange can be important to the vitality of the professionals in the field. In addition, the family benefits from the shared expertise of the two professionals. Under their careful guidance and with the benefit of their experience, the family has the opportunity for growth with new insights.

SYSTEMS THEORY

The systems theory underlies family approaches (Minuchin, 1985) and informs the work of the family consultant. In systems theory, the behavior of any family member is understood in the context of the others in the family. The situation in which a behavior occurs increases the family consultant's understanding. The consultant looks at family rules that are followed; family roles that have been assigned and are taken; and the various relationships that are held (Fine, 1984).

All behavior within the system, whether it be healthy or unhealthy, is understood within the systems framework as behavior within a given context. French (1977) defines the system as one composed of a set of elements and a set of rules that determine the relationships. The function of the system is such that the whole is greater than the sum of its parts. Systems theory maintains that any system is an organized whole with interdependent parts. Each individual is part of an organized system.

Patterns of behavior and communication are circular in the system. Behavior and communication may be exhibited by one individual in the system and then are responded to by another, or by many others in the system. Behavior and communication are not presented in a void. So, behavior, communication, and responses to them eventually become patterns of interaction between the system members. It is these patterns that develop over time that result in a set of rules for the members of the system. These rules are what govern the organization within the system—organization that is either healthy or unhealthy.

Homeostasis exists within a system; it promotes and maintains the stability of the created patterns. We then have a self-regulating behavioral style (Minuchin, 1985). The homeostatic qualities often resist change in the system (Fine, 1984). This quality is a kind of balance which assists the system in operating in a predictable manner. In a family, the members know what to expect, for example, when father drinks, or when a given child acts out. The family knows how all members will behave around the table at family meal time and who will select the television programs. Everyone in the family knows these situations, because they have been functioning as a system where one behavior is conditioned by another.

Systems consultation is described by Wynne, Weber, and McDaniel (1986) as an application of the systems concepts and the principles of consultation to work with families. Systems consultation, then, provides a strategic and appropriate framework for identifying problems within family therapy. It also allows professionals to consider options for action.

Family systems are complex. They are composed of subsystems which create a dynamic, making each family unique as a system. Subsystems in families are usually composed of parents and children. Often, a subsystem will contain a parent and one or more children. We identify the children as a subsystem and the parents become another. In any one family, we may have several subsystems. The boundaries between the subsystems are clear. The crossing of these boundaries is regulated by the family's rules. The rules protect the balance of the family system, resulting in either a healthy or unhealthy balance. Everyone in the family system can depend on the adherence to the rules, which result in consistency and reliability in the behavior of all.

Viewing the family as an organized system necessitates an understanding of the individual as a contributing member of this system. This results in a more comprehensive view of the individual. The perception is contextual. The individual is a part of the process that creates and maintains the patterns which regulate the behavior of the whole system (Minuchin, 1985). The process of causality is circular in the systemic viewpoint (Fine and Holt, 1983). Each member influences the others and reciprocally is influenced by the others. What one person in the system does structures the behavior of the others in the system (Gazda, 1984). When viewing a problem behavior systemically, the therapist views the interaction of the individual within a system of which the individual is a part. The interaction is the context in which the individual is behaving. When part of the system is modified, change is likely to occur in other areas of the system as well.

Systems theory has contributed to family work by understanding the individual in relation to the family system and understanding the family in relation to the community. From this broader perspective, the identity of the family goes beyond that of the individuals and reaches out to that of the community. Individuals are seen as community beings interrelating with a variety of others, most of whom impact the behavior and communication patterns of the individual.

Family consultation can be more effective when keeping in mind the dynamics of systems. Friedman (1986) provides a well-developed description of systems thinking. He indicates that the systems approach requires a modification of our thinking away from individual rehabilitation and toward that of the organization. This systems thinking will consider the overall environment. Systems thinking, used by a consultant who also clearly circumscribes the goals of consultation, provides a helpful model when working with families. The consultant will base many decisions on the factors of systemic operation in the consultation process.

The Family Consultation Approach

Family therapists, working within the family system, become part of the system. The very nature of intervention by the therapist places the therapist in the position of entering the system. Any change to the system results in a reactionary change. This means when any new person is introduced to the system, the system adjusts in response. Family therapists, as new persons to the system, often find themselves responded to by the family in a variety of ways. At any point along the process of therapy, the therapist may feel stuck by the responses and dynamics of the family or by internal reactions the therapist has in responding to the family. It is not uncommon for a family therapist to realize therapy with the family has come to a screeching halt. Or the family therapist will sense therapy is proceeding well, yet feel the need to check perceptions. The complexity of family dynamics and interwoven themes and patterns can be confusing. Therapists benefit from confirmation that treatment is moving in a productive manner and direction (Nielsen and Kaslow, 1980). It is at these times that family consultation can be useful to a therapist, novice or veteran. In fact, periodic consultation is a good practice. Regularly scheduled consultations, even when sessions appear to be going well, can be of help. Therapists may use the time for general improvement in therapy style. The consultant may offer a new idea which brings renewed interest, impetus for further reading, or which triggers insight for the therapist. In consultation, the nature of the problem is not prejudged and offers needed objectivity. Consultation also facilitates the reframing of problems (Wynne, Weber, and McDaniel, 1986). Consultation can lead the therapist in just the right direction and may be able to encourage the therapist toward continued education in the many areas of family counseling.

Dealing with family systems is complex and can be intricate due to the interweavings of themes and relationships. Sometimes these experiences are overt and dramatic; in other situations, only an intuitive feeling tells the therapist that while exchange is occurring with the family, little is happening in treatment (Garfield and Schwoeri, 1981). A therapist can so closely align with one family member or subsystem as to be ineffective in promoting change within the whole. This happens, for example, when a therapist is active in trying to "rescue" the children in the family. The therapist has lost perspective and may not regain the necessary view of the total system. Issues can be interpreted by the therapist in ways which are potentially limiting. Thus the therapist is not seeing the systemic activity but only one small part of the activity. For example, a therapist recognizes problem behavior on the part of the child. The therapist also realizes the parents have limited parenting skills. Without assessing the possible sources for the child's behavior, the therapist ventures on a campaign of teaching parenting skills to control the behavior of the child. Yet, often, such acting out by the child is a signal of marital conflict. The therapist may have missed this possibility because, due to its being so absorbed into the system, the detouring of marital conflict through the child is very obscured. Such loss of perspective is experienced by the best of family therapists and needs to be addressed.

Consultation is a beneficial approach to providing assistance for the needs of the family therapist. The therapist can use consultation to improve therapeutic effectiveness. New information may be gained and new insights can develop which may lead to the therapist's continued growth and development. Family consultation involves the use of consultants by experienced family therapists (Nielsen and Kaslow, 1980). The consultation is brief and designed to have an impact on the system as it is composed of the family and the therapist. As soon as the therapist entered it, the family system changed. The consultant needs to recognize this placement of the therapist within the system. The consultant is in the advantageous position of stepping back to view the situation in context. Starting as an observer allows the consultant freedom to assess relationships and interactions, for example, among the therapist and family (Wynne, Weber, and McDaniel, 1986). The consultant also becomes part of the system though on a more objective scale than those who may be enmeshed.

The purpose of the consultation is to improve the quality and functioning of the system (Garfield and Schwoeri, 1981). Family consultation is an intervention in the system with the intention of leaving it in a better state of functioning. Viewing a family systemically acknowledges the complexity of the system and the relationships that are interactional and often times subtle. Family consultation must respect the system and impact it in a positive way. The consultant will build on the relationships which currently exist between therapist and family, adding to rather than distracting from them. Yet, it is clear from systems theory concepts that the consultant is affected by the family–therapist system. The consultant needs to join with the members of the system for the purpose of the consultation, then disengage from the system. This process is managed through a variety of models of consultation.

Models

In one common approach the consultant works with the therapist (Garfield and Schwoeri, 1981; Nielsen and Kaslow, 1980) as a peer. The consultant is asked to provide an experience of self-examination for the therapist. For example, the therapist may have become aligned primarily with one member of the family, such as the mother, and is unable to join with the entire family as a system. When the therapist joins with the individual member exclusively, the systemic approach is abandoned. (This is not to be confused with siding with a member temporarily as a technique for the benefit of the entire system.)

Verification of diagnosis and/or treatment are also needs the therapist may find answered in consultation. Perception checks are useful. An outside party can bring objectivity, clarity, and another view to the situation. Nielsen and Kaslow (1980) describe this type of collegial arrangement in three different settings. One setting is among peers in an agency, clinic, or private practice. Here, the collegial relationship is with those with whom the therapist is working. The therapist's peer becomes the consultant. In another setting, an outside consultant is called in for special help. This occurs when the therapist is in solo practice or when the peer relationship may not lend itself to a collegial consultation, as when the colleague is not trained in family work and does not understand systems theory, or when there is too much tension between the colleagues or within one colleague. The third setting is the academic or training environment. A respected visiting therapist is asked to consult on a specific case or treatment issue. The case has been conducted by a therapist in a nearby practice, and the therapist and family have agreed to meet with the consultant over a designated period of time, usually one or two days. The family session is viewed by professionals attending the training program. Skills and techniques are exemplified and later discussed. Another approach to the training model is to focus on a particular treatment issue, such as families and alcoholism or abusing families. The consultant may choose any of these models and provide a comprehensive service. The choice, as with all consultation programs, is based on the needs of the consultee(s).

Several procedures may be useful in conducting family consultations. The approach chosen depends on the needs of the therapist, the availability of time and equipment, the setting, and the style of consultation comfortable to the consultant. The possibilities range from simple and brief to elaborate and involved. First, the consultant may simply discuss the experience of therapy with the therapist. The therapist has the opportunity to describe the direction therapy has taken and discuss interactions and questions which have arisen. The consultant helps by developing questions and offering feedback regarding observations. The role of the consultant in this discussion-oriented approach is one of resource for ideas or approaches, sounding board, interpreter, challenger, and stimulator. This is often the most convenient approach between colleagues and/or co-workers. It requires little prior preparation and organization aside from scheduling time between the two professionals.

Another approach to family consultation involves audio- or videotaping. This procedure requires some additional preparation between professionals. It also takes more time and demands more attention to the issues of trust between the professionals. Permission from the family to use the tapes is also necessary. All this coordination may pay off in increased accuracy in the consultation process. Taping offers a clearer view of the family and the therapy process, from which, the consultant can develop a diagnostic picture. However, since there are so many procedures to follow in setting up this type of consultation, the consultant's assistance is important. It is within the role of the consultant to assist the therapist in the procedures, ensuring that the session runs smoothly. In addition, the consultant helps with issues of trust. Introducing taping to the family presents a new and likely threatening technique. A certain degree of trust up to this point is essential for the family to grant approval for the taping of any session. The consultant's assistance to the therapist is appropriate since the process may be new to the therapist. This type of assistance may be part of the contract between the consultant and therapist. It may also be an aspect of the relationship-building phase of the process.

When lack of time or equipment make taping difficult, the consultant may observe the session live. Live observation is time-efficient. It requires some scheduling and that notice be given to the family regarding the purpose of the observer. Yet, the time is less than that necessary in the organization of a taping session. Subtle interchanges or the overall tone of the session may be lost on a tape but are more readily seen when the consultant is present. The consultant may be viewed as an intruder, however, at least initially. This experience can be avoided if the consultant is able to observe through a one-way mirror. In either case, the role the consultant plays is the same as in the former approaches. The consultant is able to take notes based on these observations. Feedback to the therapist is immediate and comes from the direct, live observations and the written notes of the consultant.

A more active consulting role is possible when the consultant participates in the session as co-therapist or sits in as a commentator. The co-therapist role is useful when the therapist has become caught in the system. The family's dynamics and games have immobilized the therapist, who is having difficulty initiating direction. The therapist has been unable to disengage sufficiently from the family to assist its progress. The goal for the co-therapist is to assist the therapist in disengaging so that the therapist can proceed with the family alone. This process empowers the therapist and sets the therapist free from the entanglement of the family. Another purpose for having a consultant as co-therapist or commentator is timing. The time may be right to try out new ideas. When the therapist is eager to experiment, it is helpful to have a trusted colleague present. It is safer to risk in this type of setting. The therapist knows that, with the consultant there, new interventions can be tried without endangerment to the family. This can be a stimulating experience for the therapist, as well as the consultant. It strengthens skills and expands techniques. Heterosexual co-therapy is recommended whenever possible (Nielsen and Kaslow, 1980). The male–female combination provides added dynamics in family work.

The consultant takes an active role in the session as a commentator. In this role the consultant makes comments during the therapy session based on observations of the family's behavior. The consultant's comments may redirect the therapy process or may reinforce the direction taken by the therapist. For this consultation approach to work well, essential ingredients include a fairly competent therapist, a trusting relationship between therapist and consultant, and respect for the therapist by the family. This model provides an excellent opportunity for therapist growth.

Planning the Consultation

Preliminary planning of the consultation will assist in making the experience a productive one. Although some approaches require less preparation than others, all consultations should be arranged and planned ahead of time. Certain considerations are important to address. These include issues relating to the family, other professionals, and the therapist's agency.

Arrangements need to be made in advance with the family. The family should be told what will take place and what their role is, if any. Especially important is informing the family as to the reason the consultation is taking place. Any member is allowed to refuse participation, yet care in explaining the event will likely reduce the chance of this kind of refusal (Nielsen and Kaslow, 1980).

The role of the therapist in planning for consultation with the family is an active one. The family's needs are important to attend to in this process. A careful description of the purpose and process defines the therapist's needs for consultation and the family's role in it. If the consultation procedure involves some of the less invasive approaches, little disturbance will be felt by the family and their role is minimal. However, it remains important for the family to know why the consultation is planned. The family can understand when a competent therapist explains the need for further training and/or an expert's opinion on diagnosis or treatment. If a trusting relationship exists between the family members and the therapist, they will more readily rely on the judgment of the therapist. Also, the family will know from the description of their role that they are involved in a training venture. This enhances the sense of their role; they are assisting the professionals in a training experience. If the family consultation is to include other professionals viewing the session, this should be explained to the family. Nielsen and Kaslow (1980) recommend that the status and roles of any observers should be clarified. The family should be invited to ask questions of the consultant and observers. Careful preparation is especially important when more invasive methods of family consultation are used, such as the consultant sitting in as observer, co-therapist, or commentator; or when observing through a one-way mirror. If the consultant is sitting in as co-therapist, the family should be informed as to the general approach the consultant may take. Some description of how the consultant will interact with the family is needed. This description is provided by the therapist prior to the consultation session. The family is also invited to feel free to interact with and question the consultant. This should all be clarified with the family members and considered part of the consultation contract. The therapist needs to be sure the family understands just how the consultation will be used.

Other arrangements are necessary for planning a family consultation. These include agency and/or supervisor approval for the consultation. For example, when a family will be interviewed by a visiting consultant, the therapist must be sure the agency or those in authority approve of the program. The agency is responsible for the treatment of patients; consequently, the agency should be involved with preliminary arrangements. Also, when there is a co-therapist as a part of the family's treatment, he or she needs to be involved in the planning and consulting experience. Hopefully the co-therapist is active from the beginning of the creation of the idea and its planning.

The Consultation Process

The actual process of consulting will involve little time. It may be brief (part of a day, as with a collegial consultation), or it may take as much as two or three days when training is involved. In any case, the time is predetermined in the planning of the consultation. Normally the family has been an ongoing case for the therapist. The therapist explains the reason(s) for the consultation to the family and obtains the family's agreement for participation. Arrangements for the family's comfort and ease are the therapist's responsibility. The therapist should be sure to greet the family on their arrival at the time of the session and be available to the family for support and any further questions and concerns which may arise. The therapist's availability may be especially necessary just prior to consultation, as anxiety may increase with anticipation.

The consultant's preparation for the interview is important to consider, especially if the consultant is involved as co-therapist or participant observer. A meeting with the therapist prior to the session offers the opportunity to establish goals for the consultation. In addition, the consultant should have access to information about the family. The consultant needs to be acquainted with the background of the members, especially regarding specific problems such as alcoholism, former therapy, previous marriages, and details about the identified patient. The consultant should also be aware of the family's socioeconomic background, ethnicity, and religious history. These factors will characterize the family experience, mores, and values.

The consultant who is informed of the multicultural dynamics of the family may avoid mistakes and misjudgments. Often a visiting consultant is unfamiliar with an area's population and its particular characteristics. Consultants should not assume they are informed but should request this kind of information. The family's values may differ from those of the consultant. For example, a Mexican American family may hold traditional values for the male and female roles in a family. The husband may expect to have a place of dominance over the wife. This traditional view may be held in regards to parenting as well. The parents may expect a position of strong authority over children. They may be less likely to accept evolving roles of women and men or to look at alternate styles of parenting. If the consultant is of another culture, for example, a white female, the consultant would be wise to consider an approach that indicates respect for the family's culture. The idea of family consultation is not to change cultural values or to conflict with them but, using the strengths of the family, to offer ways of moving beyond the problem.

Another approach to preparing for family consultation is for the consultant to avoid any in-depth discussion of the family's problem beforehand. This is the case when the consultant does not want to defuse the emotional impact of the interview (Garfield and Schwoeri, 1981). Here, the consultant prefers to see a family with little background information so that fresh impressions can be formed without filtering through the therapist's experience (Nielsen and Kaslow, 1980). The combined experiences and perceptions of the consultant and the therapist become part of the data discussed following the consultation. This approach highlights the experience of the consultant within the session. How the consultant experiences the family is a valued piece of data not diminished or filtered by the therapist's verbal or written descriptions. Frequently, an initial interview is processed by the two professionals, followed by another interview where action is taken based on the diagnostic work from the first.

Terminating Consultation

The termination process involves the consultant, the therapist, and the family. In some cases, it may involve professional observers attending the session as a part of training. After the interview, the family may be invited to remain for at least part of the analysis and discussion period which follows the interview (Nielsen and Kaslow, 1980). The family will later debrief with the therapist or, in some cases, the family may have a follow-up session with the therapist. If the family is sitting in on a discussion with therapist, consultant, and other professionals, care needs to be taken to keep the discussion focused primarily on the philosophy and techniques of the interviewer. Family dynamics should not be discussed except in relation to the approach taken by the interviewer. In this session the family is invited to ask questions and sometimes to present their perceptions of the interview. It is important to be clear about their role in the follow-up session; they are "main characters" and should be allowed an active role. When taping is used, replaying parts of the tape during the postinterview is a good idea. The use of the tape in this way may assist in highlighting points or clarifying communication patterns and family dynamics.

The model of a therapist and family follow-up interview presented by Garfield and Schwoeri (1981) provides for a session held shortly after the consultation to review the family's reaction and the consultant's recommendations. This meeting may be helpful to sort emotions stirred up during the interview. It is also a time to examine reactions and integrate understandings from the experience. The follow-up session may offer the therapist further information about the family as the therapist considers how the consultation was experienced by its members. This session has the potential of providing evaluation data helpful to the consultant. If the consultant knows this will be an approach used by the therapist, the consultant can request information about this session which is evaluative in nature. This offers the opportunity to assess the strengths and limitations of models and techniques used in the consultation. In addition, follow-up contact between the therapist and consultant allows the consultant feedback on the family's well-being and progress. This, too, is a form of feedback regarding the helpfulness of the consultation experience. Evaluation experiences of this type are useful to all parties and add a sense of accountability.

The family interview with a consultant present can be a dramatic and unusual event. The consultant may provide radical change in style, differences appealing to the family. The introduction of a new person to the system and especially one with flair can result in difficulties returning to the regular therapist. It becomes especially difficult when the consultant has been sitting in on the therapy session as co-therapist. Then two transitions need to take place: first, the transition from regular therapist to the shared therapy role with consultant as the new co-therapist. Transference of responsibility is necessary if the co-therapist is to have any impact. Second, the consultant must leave, transferring the role completely back to the regular therapist. This transition is important to the continuing therapy and must be dealt with carefully.

Transference of responsibility to the consultant can be guided by the consultant and at the same time can allow for the transference back to the therapist. Transferring responsibility to the consultant is facilitated when the consultant and family are properly prepared. Each needs to be informed about the other and their respective roles. The consultant must enter the system and bring about change in a brief period of time. This entrance is enhanced by collaborative work between therapist and consultant in the session with the family (Garfield and Schwoeri, 1981). The collaborative nature may need to be described by the two co-therapists. As the session proceeds, the consultant needs to be prepared to begin transferring authority and responsibility back to the therapist. The consultant can use the interview to clearly demonstrate the transference of responsibility and define each role. This can be done by addressing the therapist regarding the family's issues and progress. Directing concerns of this nature to the therapist makes it clear the consultant regards the therapist's knowledge of the family with respect. Stressing this respect for the therapist to the family is important. The consultant can find numerous ways of doing this. It can be done lightly and with humor or it can be displayed with intensity. Another way of assisting transference is for the consultant to take cues from the therapist which suggest the ability to defer to the authority of the therapist. Finally, the consultant may simply refer to the family's continuing work with the therapist. This assures the family that the original arrangement still holds and deters any developing fantasy ideas of the consultant becoming the new therapist.

These procedures to recognize the role of the regular therapist will facilitate the transference of responsibility and authority. It is important for the consultant to acknowledge the therapist's familiarity with and commitment to the family. Any procedures taken to ensure this will maintain the therapist's role during the visitor's interview(s). This continues the therapist's role as knowledgeable and trustworthy. The support of the therapist's role is essential to passing authority back to the therapist at the end of the family consultation interview. The consultant can acknowledge this status as temporary. This temporary position may reduce the possibility of competition between consultant and therapist. It may facilitate maximum use of the consultant's observations and recommendations by the therapist and family. Nielsen and Kaslow (1980) stress the need for the consultant to be sensitive to the problem of transfer of power. They remind the consultant to take care to avoid usurping the credibility of a fine therapist who may be perceived less glamorously simply because of close proximity. Statements of appreciation for the therapist are appropriate since it is the therapist who invited the consultant into the experience. Doing this in the presence of the family facilitates the return of responsibility for the family to the therapist.

ETHICAL CONSIDERATIONS

When a consultant dabbles in an area without adequate training, the issue is the consultant's basic competency. A consultant is usually trained in the linear, individual psychology model. The systems approach, however, necessitates retraining apart from this traditional orientation (Minuchin, 1985). The techniques used in the systems models are complex and dynamic. The family has a greater capacity than an individual to resist change, consequently, the methods of family therapy must necessarily be of greater intensity than those used with individuals (L'Abate, Ganahl, and Hansen, 1986). Approaches that surprise the family assist in moving the family structure and force the family to consider change. The sudden and unexpected may obtain results when conventional approaches do not. For example, asking a child to "pretend" to have a tantrum whenever she/he senses the parents are developing a conflict between them is a surprise intervention. It brings into the open and legitimizes the family's current functioning. The underlying message that acting-out occurs neither haphazardly nor due to the child's needs but on behalf of the marital pair moves therapy from a child-centered, behavioral base to a more global, systems-oriented focus. It forces the family to look at what is happening within the family. Since the family is systemic in nature, the change initiated by the therapist can be small and still create major changes in the family.

Additional training for the therapist may be necessary since the interventions in family therapy are less routinized and more complex than with individual therapy. The family's resistance to change necessitates that a consultant intervene with creative and, at times, dramatic and manipulative techniques (Fine and Holt, 1983). It becomes the responsibility of the professional to determine whether his/her characteristics will facilitate the effective use of these manipulative and dramatic techniques. Professional suitability is a first step, the second step is to acquire the needed educational experiences. Training, practice, and supervision of practice are necessary for responsible professional behavior and effective intervention.

Other ethical issues which need to be raised include the therapist's responsibility to avoid allowing a cooperative family being exploited. Examples are overly frequent consultant interventions with the same family for the purpose of training students or as a subject case (Nielsen and Kaslow, 1980). It is advised that interventions be paced for any one family so as not to disrupt the normal therapeutic process. Another issue is raised by Fine (1984), addressed to consultants in the school setting. Consider the school consultant enlisted for the purpose of changing a child's behavior. Often school personnel, who do not understand this request, totally exclude the family and therefore eliminate any opportunity for the family to realign its relationships. What the school misses is how the behavior fits into the broader context of the family system relationships, and the purpose the behavior serves within the family. Fisher (1986) suggests an adolescent can be seen on an individual basis within the school setting and the therapist can still utilize a systems outlook. The decision for this kind of treatment needs to be preceded by a thorough study of the family. The consultant needs to be clear, when accepting the consultation role, that both parties are contracting for the same outcome. In many cases this requires extensive discussions about systems approaches at the entry level and, at times, it may require the consultant to carefully decline the invitation. When a consultant understands implications to a client the consultee does not recognize, the consultant needs to make decisions based on this awareness. In addition, when a consultant accepts work with a consultee, the consultant must be sure there is ongoing supervision. If the consultant cannot assure this, and there is no other experienced person to monitor these new approaches, the consultation should not be offered.

Ethical considerations exist around techniques in family therapy because they are often drastic and unconventional. Hughes and Falk (1981) describe reactance techniques, such as paradoxical approaches, in regards to ethical considerations consultants need to recognize. The consultant uses a paradoxical suggestion, asking the consultee to do one thing in hopes the consultee will do the opposite. This is found to be effective with those who resist change, true of many consultees. Yet the exercise of paradoxical recommendations represents nonlegitimate power over the consultee. Even though paradoxical approaches can be useful, it is highly questionable within the consultation relationship. The consultation relationship is designed to be collaborative and collegial, which leaves no room for such reactance techniques. When this type of approach is used, deception then characterizes the relationship. Wynne, Weber, and McDaniel (1986) describe the collaborative relationship between consultant and consultee as different from other professionals. Other professional relationships, such as, supervisor–supervisee, or administrator–employee imply the participants are one-up or one-down to each other. However, collaboration between peers allows for the mutual exploration of problems and implementation of solutions. Collaboration in consulting maximizes these opportunities.

The techniques used in consultation should be selected according to the consultant's ethical standards, both professional and personal. In addition, the consultant's agency can often provide directions for the ethical behavior of the consultant. Apart from these suggestions, the best guide is always to put the client population first in determining approaches used in consultation. The appropriateness of the technique to be used needs to be measured considering the setting and roles in which it will be administered. Determining intervention strategies in this way takes into account more than outcomes alone. Intervention strategies are chosen for the needs of the client population. This is the best measure of ethical decisions on the part of the consultant.

SUMMARY

This chapter has addressed family consultation as an important encounter between therapist–consultant and consultant–family. It is a process which can enhance all parties involved. The professionals in the field experience a vitality which enhances their work after leaving a training setting. The consultee–therapist receives renewal of professional skills, knowledge, and understandings. The consultant exchanges expertise and receives the opportunity to test out ideas in a variety of settings. The consultant also experiences others' approaches in the field of family therapy. And, most important, the family benefits from the shared expertise of two trained professionals. Family consultation, as in any consultation, is successful when the system prospers and grows after the consultant's departure.

REFERENCES

FINE, M. (1984). Integrating structural and strategic components in school-based intervention: Some cautions for consultants. *Techniques: A Journal for Remedial Education and Counseling*, 1, July, 44–52.

FINE, M., and HOLT, P. (1983). Intervening with school problems: A family systems perspective. *Psychology in the Schools*, 20, January, 59–66.

FISHER, L. (1986). Systems-based consultation with schools. In L. Wynne, S. McDaniel, and T. Weber (eds.), *Systems consultation: A new perspective for family therapy* (342–356). New York: The Guilford Press.

FRENCH, A. (1977). *Disturbed children and their families: Innovations in evaluation and treatment.* New York: Human Sciences Press.

FRIEDMAN, E. (1986). Emotional process in the marketplace: The family therapist as consultant with work systems. In L. Wynne, S. McDaniel, and T. Weber (eds.), *Systems consultation: A new perspective for family therapy* (398–422). New York: The Guilford Press.

GARFIELD, R., and SCHWOERI, L. (1981). A family consultation model: Breaking a therapeutic impasse. *International Journal of Family Psychiatry*, 2(3–4), 251–267.

GAZDA, S. (1984). *Group counseling: A developmental approach.* Boston: Allyn and Bacon.

HANSEN, J. and HIMES, B. (1979). Application of a cyclical diagnostic model with families. *Family Therapy*, 6, 101–107.

HUGHES, J., and FALK, R. (1981). Resistance, reactance, and consultation. *Journal of School Psychology*, 19 (2), 134–142.

L'ABATE, L., GANAHL, G., and HANSEN, J. (1986). *Methods of family therapy.* Englewood Cliffs, NJ: Prentice Hall.

MINUCHIN, P. (1985). Families and individual development: Provocations from the field of family therapy. *Child Development*, 56, 289–302.

NIELSEN, E., and KASLOW, F. (1980). Consultation in family therapy. *American Journal of Family Therapy*, 8, 35–43.

WYNNE, L., WEBER, T., and McDANIEL, S. (1986). The road from family therapy to systems consultation. In L. Wynne, S. McDaniel, and T. Weber (eds.), *Systems consultation: A new perspective for family therapy* (3–15). New York: The Guilford Press.

CHAPTER EIGHT
CONSULTATION THROUGH TRAINING AND EDUCATION

This chapter will describe consulting in the training and education environment. We will focus on the definition of consultation through training; clarification of the role which a consultant needs to employ in such an educational program; steps to take in arranging for the training program; implementing the training program; and evaluating the program. Issues which need to be considered in the use of this approach will also be discussed. Finally, a checklist is provided for the consultant to use in approaching and conducting training programs. The following case is used as an example of the kinds of programs, and therefore issues and concerns, in which a consultant may be engaged.

CASE EXAMPLE

A training presentation was about to be delivered addressing an issue directly affecting the safety and well-being of the audience. However, the consultant arrived to discover that the listeners were attending somewhat against their will or, at least, against their preference. They seemed to have little or no interest in wasting their time listening to a speaker whom they expected to have nothing to say. As if that were not enough, everyone in the room was wearing a gun!

This consultation was a training program conducted for veteran police officers who were attending a continuing education program. The entire program covered a wide variety of units of education. The officers attended training sessions in the morning, then returned to their duties for the duration of the day. They were dressed for work—meaning guns, billy clubs, badges, and so forth.

The officers were in the training program on a somewhat involuntary basis. They were required to attend for the purpose of upgrading their professional skills. They were paid to be in class, so there was incentive. In addition the training was set up within their work day, so they were working extra hours. This is a wise approach to setting times for such programs. The officers, however, had no input about the topics for the training program. The planning and organization were done by others, and the officers had to rely on them for a program of relevance. In many cases, the officers would have rather been on duty. Going back to the classroom for further training is not easy for members of the police force who have come to rely on the "regs" for determining behavior. The training may be seen as upsetting an otherwise smooth routine. This attitude is not uncommon for many trainees in similar situations.

The organization of this program did not lend to relationship building between the officers and the consultant. The program had different trainers every day and the topics varied with the trainers. Consequently, the officers were experiencing a new face, a new topic, and likely a new approach each day. They did not easily invest in this process, knowing the trainer would be gone tomorrow and another would take his place. Thus their expressions of suspicion and even hostility were quite understandable.

Consultation through training is one of the most difficult situations a consultant encounters. This is because the time frame for joining with the consultees, for establishing a sense of trust and safety, and for building relationships is limited. It sometimes feels like a trade-off between connecting with consultees and providing the training. As consultants, we cannot separate the two. If we are just trainers, we may not need to attend to the interpersonal issues. As consultants, however, we bring a much fuller sense of the concerns with us to the training program.

TRAINING AND EDUCATION

In training and educational consulting, the consultant is invited into the role as educator. The consultant is to impart educational material to a staff or, more often, part of a staff (Imber-Black, 1986). The consultant is seen as having knowledge from which the staff can benefit and is asked to create a formal, educational program (Fisher, 1986). This may happen in two ways. First, the consultant may be contracting an ongoing consultation program which involves individual and/or group consultation. The consultant, in agreement with the contracting consultee(s), realizes the need for a training package. This training package is presented in conjunction with the ongoing consultation. The educational portion of the program compliments the consultation. It is frequently offered early in the consultation process and considered part of the intervention. Following the training program, the consultant has the opportunity to follow through with the consultees in an individual or a group consultation approach. The training and education model is one for the consultant to consider. Like so many other models, it may be most effective when used in conjunction with other models.

This training component within a broader consultation program is found in a variety of consultation situations. One such situation is a teacher consultation program where behavior modification concepts are taught in training sessions at the beginning of the consultation. Formal training using lectures, films, videotapes, handouts, and homework assignments is provided to introduce the basic understanding of behavior change. These sessions are followed by small group consultation experiences where consultants work with the consultees to develop skills in behavior change within the classroom (Hansen, 1977). The small groups are used to advise, guide, support, and share behavior-change programs the teachers are implementing in their classrooms. Without the training module, the consultant would have spent a great deal of time in small groups trying to instruct. The type of material did not lend itself to a small group format. The classroom presentation of material was the best model for this situation.

The two models of training and consulting work well in parent consultation programs. A training program for parents was offered through a mental health center teaching parents skills in interpersonal communication and in behavior modification (Himes and Hansen, unpublished). The program integrated teaching and consulting within each session. During each session, the parents were introduced to new material in an informal teaching style. The consultant then processed this material in such a way the parents were encouraged to apply it to situations at home. In this particular situation, it was best to introduce the educational material slowly and permit time to react, try out, and integrate the material. A variety of useful styles are possible when combining the educational component with consultation. It may very well be that it is ideal to pair education with consultation. Alone, education and training have no component with which to continue with the consultees. In-service training is often a valuable springboard for consultation (Conoley and Conoley, 1982). However, it is important to recognize that in-service training and workshop educational programs can be approached as a trainer or as consultant. These roles will be addressed and differentiated as we proceed.

A second approach to consultation through training and education involves the primary focus on training and education. In this model, the consultant is an in-service trainer in a workshop or training session without the accompanying consultation time. The consultant gives training that matches the needs and interests of the agency. The case of the training program for veteran police officers is an example of this model. This type of approach deserves some attention because, although it is used frequently by consultants, it is infrequently developed in research. Despite all the times a consultant may conduct a workshop, we have precious little research from which to learn about this approach. The concern with this type of approach is that, without follow-up consultation, significant behavior changes may not occur. Conoley and Conoley (1982) suggest this model be seen as a means to an end, not an end. Therefore, this chapter will address this model and provide ideas as to its integration along with the consultation model.

THE CONSULTANT AS TRAINER

The consultant is a trainer, but without abandoning consulting skills. That is, even though the consultant is taking on a new and somewhat different role, the consultant does not lose the perspective of a consultant. Bellman (1983) has shown us how the two roles are different in terms of expectations or orientations. He suggests the perspectives of the trainer may impede our effectiveness as consultants. It seems a trainer is focused on what happens in the workshop rather than in the workplace. That is, the trainer is likely to spend time preparing for a well-organized program which may be held in a site away from the consultees' center of work. Consequently, the trainer has limited knowledge of what is happening in the workplace or how the consultees experience it. The trainer's reality is focused on the material and the knowledge the trainer has of people. The consultant goes beyond this type of preparation to investigating the experiences of the consultees at their place of work: the tasks, duties, responsibilities, financial concerns, work priorities, various levels of communication, and other specifics unique to the work setting. The work setting and the agency as a system are a continued focus for the consultant. The consultant has commitment to the agency and will be cognizant of the impact of the training program on the system, as well as on individuals.

The trainer may bring a narrow focus to the workshop which prevents the trainer from identifying with and applying issues of business.

This results in misplaced priorities—no doubt what occurred in the police training program cited above. In that case, the consultant instructed in the area of communications as applied to family dynamics. These family dynamics are important for police officers to recognize when intervening in domestic disputes. It was this process in which the consultant, with good intentions, was involved in training the police officers. The consultant moved through the material with clarity and a single-minded focus. When the moment came to establish a practical application to this material, volunteers were ready to role play. Since this was the first role play, and assistance seemed called for, the consultant coached the actor in the intervention of a scene between the "husband" and one police officer, while the "wife" was allegedly in the kitchen talking to the police officer's partner. The recommendation given to the police officer, who was earnestly working with the concepts being taught, was for the officer to be aware of his nonverbal messages. In addition, the officer was encouraged to diminish the difference between his role as a representative of the police force and that of the husband who, only moments before, had exhibited the fury of his temper. The consultant, in all intensity and investment in perceptions, demonstrated the action for the police officer. In response, the police officer taught the consultant an unforgettable lesson. The police officer, who had been sitting during the entire experience, stood up—all six feet four inches of him. As he rose, the officer exhibited his regalia and explained how his pistol would have been inches away from the angered husband had he followed the consultant's directions. As if that were not enough to paint the picture, he proceeded to describe the acute danger each officer faced when responding to domestic dispute calls. The descriptions were somehow far more vivid than all the reading the consultant had done on the topic. The entire focus of the workshop changed as a result of this gentle, but direct, confrontation. This example may demonstrate the problem we, as consultants, have when we emphasize the trainer role. We tend to not acknowledge the reality of what is happening in the workplace.

When the consultant is present in the workplace, the training can be done in a more complete context. The inside consultant, or the outside consultant who spends a good deal of time in the setting, will experience the crises, the deadlines, the tensions. Often the consultant needs to make on-the-spot decisions. The trainer has the luxury of coming into a setting, often elsewhere than the actual work setting, with a great deal of preparation time. What the trainer has to say is planned. The trainer relies on what is brought to the training session and often does no more than field questions from the people attending. The trainer does not have the benefit of using the strengths of the participants in dealing with issues, because the trainer lacks familiarity with them. The trainer's approach is planned, whereas the consultant will more than likely respond spontaneously (Bellman, 1983; Conoley and Conoley, 1982) using the teachable moment.

A consultant who provides training sessions will be inclined to look at issues within a system of an organization. Too frequently, a trainer who is not using the broad spectrum of consulting skills will appear to provide solutions to independent problems without looking at what these solutions will create in the total system (Fisher, 1986; Kurpius, 1985). The consultant will ask questions to assist participants in searching for manageable answers. Fewer answers and more questions will be raised (Bellman, 1983). The consultant will be aware the participants have a great deal of expertise of their own; faith in the consultee's abilities is exhibited by the consultant.

All too often a trainer appears on the doorstep of the workshop setting very ready to take charge. This is true when the trainer has come knowing what is to be said, knowing the questions, and knowing the answers. When we are that set on what will take place, however, we are no longer open to what the consultees may offer, to different realities from those we have imagined true for the consultees. For example, the consultant's surprise in the police training program existed because the officer presented a reality of the job which was missed by the consultant. The consultant responded with openness to the new perspective and was willing to relinquish control over the session for the benefit of the learning process. It is true the consultant does not have all the answers, and many opportunities exist for collaborative experiences between the consultees and consultant. In this role, the consultant–trainer will offer adequate structure to learn and listen to the consultees (Hansen and Himes, 1977). The consultant–trainer will teach in workshops with a flexible format and have a body of preplanned information (Conoley and Conoley, 1982). The consultant–trainer will rely on the consultees' issues to move and guide direction and to place emphasis.

We need to view the larger picture of the system. Bellman (1983) suggests focusing on the larger organization rather than just the individuals within the institution. This broader picture of the organization allows us to understand that everyone in the institution has reasons for present behavior. Change is not simple and requires a systemic understanding. The consultant will observe the institution by studying the physical setting and observe how people spend their time. They will interview employees and develop an understanding of what the institution says about its culture, and how the career path looks, and how long people stay in jobs. They will assess the communication pattern(s). This type of observation is important in the role of consultant as trainer. It provides a frame of reference from which the consultant is more than trainer; the consultant is an advocate for systemic change.

PREPLANNING FOR TRAINING PROGRAMS

A quick look at this type of program may suggest it saves time for the consultant. This is true when the outside consultant is seldom at the work-site, while the inside consultant may perceive this as an easy programming approach. It may be seen as saving consultant time. The reality is that a good deal of time is spent in preparation for training programs. This is true for both external and internal consultants. However, how the consultants spend their time in the preplanning can be quite different. These differences will be explored by addressing the separate positions of the consultant–trainer external to the agency and the internal consultant–trainer.

Consultant Trainers External to the Agency

Planning for the specific topic. The wise consultant will approach the initial session with an openness to the needs of the consultees and with few preconceptions. The temptation is to jump to a solution, a model, a theory, and sometimes even a gimmick which the consultant has used before. However, the consultant must not meet with the consultee(s) thinking, "I know just what you need," "I have just the right approach." The consultant may arrive at just the right approach, but this should be done by joining with the consultee(s) and exploring the concern together (Hansen and Himes, 1977). The process is a collaborative one.

Fisher (1986) suggests that entering a system as an outside consultant places you in the position of being the expert. It is not uncommon for staff to feel competitive toward you. This competition may even be somewhat natural when, for example, the administration is sending messages about the inadequacy of the staff. If the staff is lacking in some area, the presence of an outside consultant will only highlight this. Resistance may result. Katz (1984) speaks of hostility on the part of the participants. It becomes important that the consultant understands some of this reaction, respects where the consultees may have developed these feelings, and works collaboratively and effectively in the task of training.

This initial activity is clearly one of exploration (Weber, McDaniel, and Wynne, 1986) where the consultant deals with the various factions and needs of the consultees. The consultant must be objective in entering the system of the agency, leaving personal agendas behind. Since there is a need to develop a healthy contract with an agency, the consultant needs to be prepared to explore with the consultees, for the purposes of meeting their goals and needs. The consultant is not free to do whatever seems right but must be sensitive to this new territory and willing to explore the many possibilities with the consultees.

The first step is to discover what the agency is all about. If you are a consultant from within and providing a training program for your agency, knowledge of your agency is far more available. However, the external consultant must explore and inform him or herself. The outside consultant needs to listen to the consultee(s) talk about goals and purposes. It is useful to hear the passions and disappointments of the people who have initiated the request for consultation. The consultant must recognize where the consultees fit in the hierarchy of the institution, knowing this can be helpful in assessing their request and their concerns. For example, some requests will come from administrators who are asking for consultation to fulfill state requirements or funding requirements. This may result in a distinct lack of investment on the part of the administrators for the consultation program.

The consultant's assessment of the agency administration and organization will allow the consultant to determine who are key personnel with whom to meet. As a consultant external to the institution, distance may be a factor in meeting with personnel. It is important, however, to make every effort to meet people before the consultation and, if possible, see the work setting. If this is impossible, a telephone conference can be set up to assist in gathering information. Whichever approach is used the consultant needs to be prepared with a process for gathering information. Questions specific to the history and needs of the agency are useful. If there is a crisis concern, the background of the crisis should be developed. Help the consultees to describe with incidents, quotes, file notes, and other factual and experiential data. Do not assume the consultees understand the concern completely and with much perspective. Your questions will not only assist you and the process of collaboration, but the consultees as well.

An excellent approach to gathering data is to develop a needs assessment. This is very helpful when an agency has only a general idea of needs. The assessment can be developed to offer a wide range of ideas, concerns, and questions. The responses from the staff will assist in selecting key areas which are of concern to the employees. The assessment approach is particularly useful when an area of concern has been identified. The consultants can use the written needs assessment to break a particular topic area into its component parts (Conoley and Conoley, 1982). This approach to consultant planning gives some planning guidance. It tends to reveal any discrepancies which exist, such as between administrators who are pressured to have programs to fulfill state regulations and other staff who want to have programs offering something practical and tangible to assist them in their on-the-job tasks. For example, funding sources require counseling components of organizations to have in-service training for the counselors. The administrator may not know just what needs the counselor has on a client-to-client basis. The counselors, however, could describe this with quite some detail. They know what problems they are having and what assistance they need. They can describe, for example, the types of cases, the particular problems at a particular stage, concerns about follow-up, questions about referrals, and management of crises. In addition, the counselor knows individual needs, fears, and inadequacies which a training program can begin to address. Hearing from the counselors makes a great deal of sense in planning the consultation program.

The needs assessment offers guidance in planning the session. The consultant, however, must also look beyond the information offered in the needs assessment. The consultant must recognize any significant differences between administration and other employees and meet a balance between these areas of need. Fisher (1986) suggests the consultant may be used by one group to ally against an antagonist who could be an administrator or another subgroup. If the discrepance is too wide or it seems the consultant is being asked to promote someone's personal concerns which do not address those of the agency, the consultant should raise this issue. If it is possible to resolve the discrepancy, the program will be much more applicable and useful. Should the consultant discover the program is evolving as a personal statement from just one person, or one faction of the organization, the consultant should decline to be involved.

Any method of involving participants in the planning of the program will increase the sense of personal commitment. Needs assessments are one way. Another is to personally meet with the staff and discuss concerns in an informal way. Other methods may be created by the consultant, who knows personal enthusiasm and investment in the in-service training will promote success of the consultation program.

Contracting.   Contracting may be a more critical issue for the outside consultant than the consultant training from within the agency. However, the internal consultant may wish to develop a contract as well. Potential problems and misunderstandings can be avoided by spelling out in writing what is expected of both the consultant and consultees in the implementation of the program (Stewart and Medway, 1978). The external consultant usually has two main areas of concern in the written contract. These are the explanation of the specific topic of consultation and the consulting fee. When the consultant describes the topic of the program, the time and location can also be discussed. The consultant and consultees will have already arrived at a date and time for the consultation prior to contract writing, so this can simply be stated. The location and all the associated factors which accompany this issue, should be done by the consultees. It is the consultant's place to present this task with clarity to the consultees during the preplanning phase. Details such as the following should all be part of the preplanning: comfortable and convenient space; freeing of employee time for the program; selecting a time when all employees can attend without undue inconvenience; materials which may be duplicated at the agency's expense (sometimes this is contracted as an expense of the consultant); these they simply need to be stated in the written contract for a reminder and/or clarification.

The second area of contracting is that of the consulting fee. This is an issue peculiar to the outside consultant, as it is rare the inside consultant needs to deal with a fee. The fee, like the preliminary plans, needs to be discussed and agreed upon before the contract letter is scripted. The consultant needs to have a clear statement of the remuneration, per day, per hour, or for the total program. Frequently, the organization the consultant represents has a standard fee which defines the amount. If, however, the consultant is independent, and/or this is a consultation program which cannot be determined by former practice, there are a few steps to take in forming the fee. One initial step is to inquire about agency ability to pay. Frequently, the agency is being funded to have in-service programs, such as by government funding. Their costs may already be established. In these cases, little negotiation may be possible. Other times, such as in the case of the police training program, you may be hired to conduct a part of a total program. This program was held through the police academy at the local community college. The fee was contracted with the academy, and the consultant received the standard remuneration for guest speakers.

The second step to consider in establishing a fee is whether the participants have the capacity to pay a fee. This may be possible when, for example, a school district organizes a teacher in-service training program. Teachers volunteer to participate in the sessions, pay a fee to the consultant and, in return, the school offers the teacher a continuing education unit which is applied toward contracting their salary. The agreement to give continuing education units is set between consultant and administration in the preplanning. This approach meets needs of all involved. The administration arranges for training in areas of concern for the teachers. The teacher receives credit for attendance which will impact salary ranking. The consultant is reimbursed for the training program. This is a good approach to contracting which takes everyone's needs into consideration.

A third possibility for the consultant to consider is a contract without a fee. At first glimpse this may not seem attractive to the consultant. However, there are many agencies which are providing much-needed services in nonprofit organizations, such as the YMCA or YWCA, childrens' summer camps, church programs, Planned Parenthood, city or town programs like recreational programs, parent groups within schools, like the PTA, and many other organizations. These agencies need training and education just as much as others. Some of these agencies have funds in their budgets for consulting fees, others do not. Many consultants will look for nonprofit organizations to which they can donate their services on a regular basis. Besides the genuine good feeling of doing a service for others, this approach offers the consultant visibility which may lead to other programs. This result is unpredictable and should not be the motivation. Yet, it is possible that someone in the nonprofit organization is a part of—or knows someone who is connected to—another organization where consultation is also needed. And so it goes. The visibility is matched by credibility. A free workshop in an organization which has no ability to pay could lead to referrals. Personal references are the best way to continue in the consulting business. Also, a free or low-cost workshop with an agency with the capacity to pay may give the consultant credibility with that agency. Consequently, the agency may contract for further consultation, either continued training programs or ongoing consultation.

The written contract is a clear summary statement describing the conditions of the consultation training. It should be written by the consultant and sent to the consultee with whom the negotiations were made, with copies sent to any other pertinent group(s). The consultant should be sure to know who needs to receive copies of the contract. The contract is mailed well in advance of the actual training program. This will allow time for any response or clarification which may occur. However, if the contract is written based on careful planning, the written contract is a process after-the-fact.

Consultant Trainers Internal to the Agency

Internal consultants have different needs than those outside the agency. They do not need to contract for a fee due to the fact that they are employees within the institution, such as a counselor within a program offering counseling, or a school psychologist within a school system. However, they may need to contract for a different time schedule or a different role definition. Also, information regarding the institution is readily at hand. The internal consultant will need to establish time to consider what is already known and gain some objective on this understanding. It is wise if the consultant can step back and view the institution systemically rather than as an agency made up of individuals. Issues the inside consultant must attend to are: topics for consultation and consultant credibility; arrangement of time and space for the consultation training; and participation in the training program.

Topics for consultation and consultant credibility.   The objectivity obtained in considering the needs of the agency may assist the inside consultant in determining topics. Often, the inside consultant wishes to present a training program filling a need perceived by the consultant. In other cases, the request may come from a colleague or the administration. It is possible the inside consultant has had specific training and/or experience outside the agency. The consultant is then in the situation of being able to teach colleagues, thereby sharing the wealth. In any case, it makes sense for the consultant to use the needs assessment approach described above to have input from the potential participants. It is always a wise move to use this type of approach because the participants have been asked to be a part of the planning. Their investment can help the overall process, and their input is useful. For example, it is not unusual for the consultant within a school to instruct in the training program using the teachers' descriptions and phrases found in the needs assessments. This allows the words of the teachers and possibly some examples of the classroom to be demonstrations in the training. This style is much more effective and real than bringing something which may relate to the topic but not to the people. The needs assessment is always a good reference for future training programs. What is not addressed in the present program can be considered for another time.

Consultant credibility is linked with the topic in that the consultant must be credible in the area to be taught. This type of credibility is slowly established and is usually well earned. Word-of-mouth is the most effective way of letting one's professional expertise be known. Colleagues are typically slow to acknowledge the expertise of another. Respect for the consultant will likely facilitate the interest in working with the consultant. Also, the way the consultant chooses to share the information with others impacts on the acceptance of the consultant. Acceptance is more probable when the consultant shares as an equal. For example, when a consultant returns to the place of work from an outside conference, training program, or class, the consultant may wish to share the experience. How this sharing is done may impact on whether or not credibility begins to be established. The formality or informality, the aggressiveness, the elitist attitude, the genuine care about the agency and colleagues, the ability to include others in one's enthusiasm for the material all have a great deal to do with the receptiveness of the consultant's colleagues and administration.

Arrangement of Time and Space for the Consultation

It is most likely the inside consultant will be responsible for making the arrangements for the consultation. In ideal situations, a committee may be formed to assist, or other individuals will facilitate these arrangements under the direction of the consultant. The process of these arrangements is not difficult, but it is often tedious. The process needs to be handled with attention to the way the system works. For example, the inside consultant will know who to speak to first, even as a figurehead, before going to the person(s) who can actually help get the task done. Be sure to follow the procedures respectfully, so as not to "step on any toes." Being a part of the system means the inside consultant has knowledge of how things work. There are built-in guidelines which, although unwritten, are clear enough to facilitate the work of the consultant.

The arrangement of time for the training program may actually take more time than any other single factor. It presents itself as a headache for the consultant who needs to please a number of groups. Yet, the effort taken to select the best time for all is beneficial. Attendance may hinge on the time selected, and the general feeling about attending can be impacted by it. The first thing a consultant needs to do is find out what the possibilities are for arranging time. This will vary widely. In some agencies, the time will be dependent on the size of the agency. For example, when there are few staff persons to do the work in a eight-hour day, it becomes difficult to free up time within the working day. Additional time in the evening or on a Saturday may be necessary. This will be attractive only if the payoffs are beneficial to the participants. Payoffs are entirely possible. Beyond the benefits of the training to the individual, it is possible the agency can provide pay or compensation time for the training hours. Other circumstances are possible in larger institutions. For example, two training programs can be offered so one group is trained while another is covering the workload of the first. Schools, however, have an entirely different situation. This is often the most problematic arrangement of time an inside consultant may deal with.

The inside consultant within a school system has the contract of the teachers' union to appreciate. This is often very restrictive in terms of establishing time outside the teaching day for in-service programs. Even an hour before school or after school is unlikely because of the contract. Any time such as before or after the school day, during the evening, or on Saturday must be voluntary. Although voluntary attendance is highly desirable, it may not prove to gather the number of teachers a consultant would hope for a training program. An added problem is that volunteers who choose to attend such a program on top of their teaching hours could be hassled by the union. Pressure may be placed on them to not do more than is required by the contract for the purposes of future contracting. These are real concerns which may impede attendance and/or attitude. The inside consultant seems to have more of this type of problem than the outside consultant, at least until credibility is established. Perhaps the most convenient approach to selecting time is to use the already-established time period of conference days. Most schools have a few conference or in-service days set aside from the beginning of the year. District administrators have established these as paid conference days for the benefit of training the teachers. These are scheduled early, so the consultant would need to claim that time well in advance. This may be a drawback when the consultant wants to address a relevant issue which has surfaced as the school year has progressed. If the conference time is already distributed, the consultant only has the choice of waiting another year, which is hardly a desirable situation for timely issues. When consultant credibility, administration awareness, and teachers' willingness to volunteer begins to change, the situation of establishing time will become much easier for the consultant within schools.

An issue similar to time arrangement is the obtaining of space for the training program. Like the issue of time, finding space varies from agency to agency. Some agencies have rooms specifically for conferences, meetings, and the like, which are perfectly suited for in-service training because they have been designed for this. They come equipped with audio-video capacities and a place for the coffeepot. Other agencies have to scramble for space which may prove to be less-than-satisfactory for such an occasion. Unfortunately, the result is the consultant takes what there is and makes due.

Participation in the consultation training. The issue of participants in the training is tangential to those described above. Basically, the issue revolves around the voluntariness and involuntariness of the participants. We recognize this is not an either/or situation. Participants who are not initially inclined to attend a session can be coaxed—some would say bribed. If inducements are enough to make it worthwhile, the participants will be more voluntary. We have come to expect such reinforcements in our world of work. These tangible rewards should never preclude the quality of the program. Ultimately, this is the best reward for active attendance. Participants who are initially inclined to attend, could change their voluntary status to involuntary, given certain factors. The lack of quality in the program, the presenter's style, or a change in focus or topic may occur resulting in consultee disappointment. If the participant agrees to attend with a certain idea about the program and this is changed, the participant has the right to become upset. Voluntary attendance scheduled at times suited to the participants is usually the optimal choice for the internal consultant (Conoley and Conoley, 1982). Keeping the needs of the consultees in mind will guide the consultant in choosing options. Also keep in mind that you may be better off with a small, motivated group of people who are happy with the program and the way it was established. Future programs are more likely with this type of result.

IMPLEMENTATION

Effective implementation of the consultation training program is dependent on how the consultant connects with the consultees. There is less time for this type of connecting in a training program than in a longer-term consultation program. In programs with more time, the consultant also has the advantage of more time for diagnosis, observation, questioning, and general assessment. Consequently, when the contract is written, the consultant is ready to begin with a one-shot approach. This is a distinct disadvantage when there is no other consultation to continue after the workshop is completed. This fact should be remembered by the consultant, and it can guide the consultant in the implementation. It may guide the consultant away from material which is too complex or confusing, from moving too quickly, and from being careless because the consultant remains with the consultees for such a short time.

Planning

The consultant needs to block out a significant period of time for preparation of the training. Once the preplanning is done, the consultant must be intentional about providing quality material. Care should be taken to be clear about what is being communicated. Integrate a variety of methods of teaching with the recognition that there are a variety of ways of learning. For example, many people are assisted with written material, either on the chalkboard or in handouts. They retain information better when they can follow along or see things laid out in an outline form. Outlining the program for the participants is a good way of informing them about their activity with you. This offers the consultees a type of a road map which is a good way of keeping participants with you. In addition to providing an outline, or as a part of the outline, the consultant can provide consultation objectives. These goals and purposes for the program help to guide the participants in what they may be looking for in the consultation. Other consultees are assisted by audio-visual aids. Using the right film may demonstrate a point you are trying to make far better than continuing a lecture. Others can learn best when involved in experiential activities, such as role plays. None of these ideas are gimmicks. They are teaching approaches based on different kinds of learning styles. Use them with careful planning and with intentional organization.

Conducting the Session

The planning must be well developed, however, it need not be overly structured. Flexibility will allow the consultant to adjust the material to the needs, ideas, and questions of the consultees. A sense of good timing becomes part of this approach as well. The consultant can "read" the consultees to evaluate their needs. It may be that an unscheduled break is called for or the abandonment of some of the material, or the change of approach will be necessary. These useful alterations in the program cannot be foreseen by the consultant. If the consultant is inflexible, the needed changes as well as integration of consultee involvement is not possible. For example, when a group of enthusiastic consultees have had the opportunity to sink their teeth into a bulk of the material, they are ready and able to process the material in a group discussion which the consultant had not planned. The inflexible consultant will not permit this change since it will disrupt the schedule and carefully made plans. It is wise for the consultant to allow a good discussion to continue beyond the scheduled time limit when it is beneficial to the consultees as a whole. This is true, even if the consultant wanted to move on to some other planned activity or if the consultant had plans for discussion later. The time is right for this activity to be encouraged. Later, the group may have lost their investment. Another approach may not capture their involvement. The consultant needs to be flexible enough to adjust to this new plan and to guide and support it.

The consultant will be more flexible and confident if the consultant is sure about the material. This will be conveyed to the consultees when the consultant has command of the material and presents it in styles which enhance the learning process. Give yourself sufficient time to prepare; plan for teaching approaches; arrange for any needed audio-visual equipment; practice the presentation; and plan a sequencing so the teaching is varied and interesting. Sequencing the teaching activities does not mean saving the fun things for last after the boring lecture material is out of the way. It means, for example, providing a smooth sequencing of didactic, audio-visual, and experiential elements. Conoley and Conoley (1982) suggest decisions be made ahead of time for the sequencing of activities. For example, trainers can use a gradual approach to the risk level of the activities. Lectures are useful in providing a body of material and offer little or no risk for the consultee. Role-playing activities, however, which can build on the material presented earlier, involve a greater level of risk. The police training program offered didactic presentations with handouts, followed by discussion with questions encouraged, and concluded with role plays. By this time, the officers had had a number of opportunities to hear and be heard; they had observed the consultant interacting and heard the responses to concerns. This provided time to develop a sense of trust helpful for role plays which require a level of vulnerability on the part of the participants.

This type of risk-taking activity can be very productive in a training session. Participants are there to learn, which is usually done within a safe environment, and one that stretches people and requires them to move beyond where they are. Consequently, a variety of approaches may be very helpful to move the consultee in training. Conoley and Conoley (1982) indicate that training should operate a little beyond trainee comfort level. This does not give us, as consultants, an open door for experimental activities. We need to know what works, learn from our own experiences and the feedback of our trainees. We need to develop a way of judging how and if to protect consultees in training activities. Generally, we can expect that a climate of trust and acceptance within the training program, and from the preplanning work of the consultant with the agency, will give permission for consultees to attempt activities.

Staying flexible during the consultation is part of the collaborative contract. Consultants who are capable of adjusting will remain open to input and questions from consultees about the direction of the session. This is not the same as "flying by the seat of one's pants" or "winging it." These approaches do not suggest any planning or careful thought about the direction or integration of the consultees' needs. If there is no preparation, it will never all come together in the session. Planfulness can be a partner with flexibility. It is when the consultant does not plan or is too rigid with the program that opportunities for learning are missed.

EVALUATION

Formal and intentional evaluation procedures are very important to both inside and outside consultants. Consultants internal to the organization will likely need to provide a written statement about the program. Evaluation is an essential part of that. The inside consultant has many opportunities to receive verbal feedback from co-workers and should seek this type of input. However, a formal, written approach will offer concrete data on which to base the report.

The consultant external to the organization has little or no personal contact with the consultees after the training session is completed. The written evaluation is necessary feedback to the consultant. The same type of evaluation process can be followed by either the internal or external consultant.

It is wise to develop an evaluation based on the consultation goals and objectives. These are given to the consultees at the beginning of the training session and referenced frequently. When the program is constantly tied to these goals, the evaluation should be quite simple to complete as it will be familiar material. Using the same phrases and words used in the training session will help the consultees identify what is being asked in the evaluation. The written evaluation form does not need to be lengthy unless the agency requires something complex. Should this be the case, the consultant can explain the reasons for the lengthy process. When the form is brief, to the point, and designed so the consultees can answer simply, it will not take much of the consultees' time to complete. It is wise to give the form to the participants for completion just before the program is finished, as a last item. This assures the consultant a return from each participant. It is also a good time for the consultees to recall all the experiences.

Complementary to the immediate feedback of the written evaluation is a follow-up evaluation. The consultant can establish a time several weeks or a few months later to assess the level of applicability of the consultation program. This is desirable because the first evaluation cannot do this, and application is the ultimate goal of training programs. Unfortunately, this is done very infrequently. It is time consuming and quite inconvenient for a consultant external to the agency. There is a need, however, and all consultants are encouraged to proceed with such responsible endeavors.

There are other possibilities for evaluation. The consultant can be creative and plan evaluative experiences which best fit the type of program, location, staff, and circumstance of each consultation. For example, an consultant was successful in acquiring agency help from employees in the planning stage. A committee of people who were committed to the idea of training, and to the issues, were involved in establishing goals for the program. Activities and approaches were discussed within the committee meetings, which the consultant attended. Thus, this committee had the potential of being a continued resource to the consultant. The consultant met with the committee eight weeks later to discuss observations made by the committee regarding applicability of the training program. In some cases, data other than verbal feedback can be gathered in this follow-up (Hansen, 1977). Consultants are encouraged to evaluate consultation programs (Gallessich, 1982; Bardon, 1985) and most frequently measure client population with whom the consultees have been working. However, we are able to move in yet another direction. We can assess the changes that occur in the consultees themselves (Bardon, 1985). This would include the behavior, attitudes, feelings, and intentions of the consultees. These aspects of the consultee approaches to clients are all directly influenced by consulting programs which are educationally oriented. Bardon suggests we need to observe what happens to consultees first.

Exiting. The evaluation is likely to be the outside consultant's last face-to-face activity with the consultees. An exception is when the training consultant will be following up with consultation and/or a follow-up evaluation is established to assess the application of the consultation. A report is usually written. However, this is likely to be mailed to the contacting party. Consequently, as the consultees submit their evaluations at the conclusion of the training program, the consultant is exiting. This is typically done with a brief statement of pleasure and/or delight in being able to join with this group for the training experience. Since the training program without further consultation is brief, the exit statement calls for the same. Any more would be less than graceful.

ISSUES

There are many considerations to observe when planning the involvement of a training program. These include the concern of training with no follow-up consultation, ethical considerations, and multicultural concerns.

Training with No Follow-Up Consultation

When consultation does not follow training, the consultant has no way of continuing with the consultees. The training is a one-shot approach which may or may not be effective on a long-term basis. Stein (1975) suggests that brief workshop or seminar format methods of teaching are inadequate in instructing principles and techniques of behavior modification. It may be we need to look hard at other brief training programs and be more intentional about pairing these with continued consultation. It is realistic to consider the likelihood that a number of participants in a workshop cannot follow through with ideas presented on their own. Many would need the continued support, encouragement, individual recommendations, observation, and specific ideas a consultant can provide in a small group or individual consultation experience following the training.

Ideally, the training is a springboard for continued work with the consultees. The training package is designed to be part of a consultation package. For example, outside consultants were employed for consultation with Headstart to conduct training programs with the teachers and staff and then provide follow-up consultation on a weekly basis. The consultants designed several day-long training sessions to be held over the academic year in areas the staff would find helpful, such as models of discipline, crisis intervention, working with parents, and helping children cope with divorce. The consultation topics were identified jointly by the staff and the consultants. When conducting the training on divorce, the consultants provided material about divorce as perceived by the adults in a family. They identified stages of divorce as experienced by the divorcing parents. They were careful to clarify the facts and myths about divorce. The focus was on the parents and the impact this separation experience had on them as well as some of the common responses to the divorce experience. A morning break was followed by a discussion period. The group was led to share fears about divorce, often based on stereotypes, sometimes based on observations of children in the program. They asked questions which surfaced during the didactic presentation earlier. Questions were fielded by the consultants who used some of their familiarity with the client population to provide well-developed responses. Consultants were intentional about keeping the focus on the consultees as often as possible. This meant encouraging the consultees to look at their own biases and prejudices which exist against divorce. In some cases, consultees needed to evaluate their personal biases and prejudices against their client population. There was a lunch break which allowed time for reflection, objectivity, and informal discussions. This type of break is often seen by consultants as a loss to the process. However, we need to recognize the many ways consultees process information and experiences. This break time is a kind of a removal from the intensity of the in-service program, yet it is precisely what many participants need. Others will not lose the ability to become involved again, they simply are refreshed and energized to return.

The afternoon session of the divorce workshop was designed to focus on the issues of divorce as they impact the child. The process having been described earlier, the picture is completed by understanding the various ways children feel, react, and learn to cope with the separation and loss they experience. Again, this session was followed by a discussion period. The consultants provided evaluations to be completed just prior to the time of leaving. This was a simple Likert-type scale designed to reflect each component of the training. The respondents merely checked the area which most closely identified their experience. An area for additional comments was provided. The consultees left with the experience in their hearts and a handout packet in their hands. The packet was given at the beginning of the session. It was printed on colorful sheets of paper associated with different topic areas of the program. A bibliography of books for divorcing adults, or adults working with divorcing parents, was provided, as well as a bibliography of books which can be read to, or by, children of divorcing parents. The bibliographies were annotated. Several of the selections were referenced in the training sessions to add familiarity to these resources.

This type of consultation package, where specific training is provided, allowed the consultants to deal directly with the issue of divorce among the client families. It facilitated the teaching of expression of feelings and biases toward divorce, and it encouraged the acceptance of the new single-parent family identity. When the teachers and staff honestly faced the issues, they were better able to assist the children and parent in doing the same. The training program initiated this process of change. The follow-up consultation, however, encouraged and gave opportunities for this change to continue.

In the cases where the consultant is not able to follow through with on-going consultation, the consultant may be able to identify someone within the institution to offer supervision. Conoley and Conoley (1982) offer the suggestion that a consultant could provide supervision by receiving tapes of attempts to apply the new skills on the job. These tapes would be reviewed by the consultant, returned in the mail, and would offer the consultee a form of supervision specific to the training objectives. The special effort this approach entailed should suggest we need to consider many possibilities for follow-up. Though cumbersome and perhaps less than perfect, such efforts can be seen as better than nothing.

Ethical Issues

What seems important for the trainer–consultant is to do training as a consultant, that is, to involve the consultees at every level: planning, joining together in the training session, and evaluation. This collaborative experience is characterized by the consultant remaining open and flexible.

Whether or not the consultant possesses established codes, published guidelines, or sanctioned directives for professional behavior, the responsibility for ethical behavior rests with the consultant. Where no such codes exist, one needs to consider the competencies the consultant brings to the program and the responsibilities taken to provide service.

Potential ethical problems which a consultant should be aware of within the consulting process include the misuse of power by the consultant. The consultant will diminish the tendency of misusing power by remaining open to the consultees' needs and by establishing a collaborative relationship with them. Also, consultants need to be clear about their roles. There may be less likelihood of confusing a consultant with a personal counselor when the consultant is involved with a brief training session, as opposed to an ongoing consultation where familiarity is increased. However, the consultant still needs to be aware some will try to put the consultant in the position of fixing everything. The wise consultant will clarify the consulting role well in advance of these problems. Another area of ethical concern is for the consultant to recognize limitations of competence and objectivity. The consultant who enjoys the ego boost of being invited into a consultation program may not consider personal strengths and limitations. It is realistic to present to consultees professional qualifications with accuracy and honesty, and to be clear as to the areas of competence. The lack of objectivity can result in a number of diagnostic problems for the consultant. The consultant must be able to determine agency readiness and need for the training programs and, consequently, for change. The consultant needs to be aware that systems have their own sense of timing and process. These should be respected while working with the organization. An associated area of concern is the tendency all helping professions have of imposing values. This is discussed in the area of multicultural concerns. It is wise to investigate the goals and purposes of the agency and consider value congruence between consultant and agency. Finally, the consultant needs to remain open to feedback and develop the capacity to self-evaluate. Evaluation should be viewed as an opportunity to grow, not unlike the training program the consultant is providing for the growth of the consultees.

The responsibility lies with the consultant for ethical behavior in the consultation. The consultant must be honest about competencies which involve the training program. The consultant must also recognize the responsibilities as consultant. Although specific guidelines do not exist, the consultant should have professional standards which direct behavior in training consultation programs.

Multicultural Concerns

The wide diversity in our communities, churches, schools, organizations, and agencies deserves respect and appreciation. The diversity is too rich to describe individual situations in this writing. However, the consultant needs to appreciate the personal backgrounds, values, and beliefs of others. One's class, ethnicity, sex, age, religion, and a number of other variables will be expressed in behavior, values, attitudes, and so forth. These areas have routinely been neglected in the training of consultants (Gibbs, 1985; Inouye and Pedersen, 1985). As a consultant is involved with the preplanning of a training program, acquiring knowledge about the multicultural factors of the consultees and clients is important. It is also helpful to use culturally appropriate intervention stategies, which will be more readily determined as the consultant becomes acquainted with the group.

Multiculturalism is becoming much more the norm in our society, and for us as consultants. Thus, cultural awareness is important. The consultant has the ethical responsibility of being aware of one's own culture, values, and beliefs, as well as understanding how these differ from others (Gibbs, 1980). The norm of multiculturalism means the consultant cannot consider the personal to be the dominant cultural style. Moving beyond the ego-centeredness of one's own culture permits the consultant to participate in a collaborative relationship with consultees. This collaboration allows the consultant to operate from a personal perspective as well as joining with the consultees who are free to own their perspectives in the consultation relationship.

CHECKLIST FOR TRAINING CONSULTANTS

The following is a checklist for the training consultant. It offers some areas of concern in establishing a responsible training program.

1. Who is making the request?
   For whom is the request being made?
   How is the problem/need described?
   Why were you asked as consultant-trainer?

2. What are the areas of the program?
    What is the history of concerns with this agency?
    Can you meet with others who will be involved?
    Is a needs assessment needed/possible?
3. Who is the consultee population?
    What is their multicultural makeup?
    Are they a voluntary consultee group?
4. Do your competencies match the request and the consultees' needs?
5. What type of fee will be established?
    What arrangements are made for space?
    What arrangements are made for time?
    What arrangements are made for materials? Who does the work? Who pays?
6. Given the topic and consultee population, what techniques can be used?
    What equipment will be needed to set up in advance?
7. What method(s) can be used for evaluation?
    Who writes the report?
    Who receives the results of consultation training?
    What method(s) can be used for self-evaluation?
8. What is the termination or exiting process with the agency?

SUMMARY

Contributions to a variety of organizations and institutions can be provided through consultation training programs (Gallessich, 1985). These can include training to schools, churches and synagogues, youth programs, college campuses, management, a variety of professional and nonprofessional groups, and so forth. Consultation training can incorporate a number of areas, such as conflict resolution, crisis intervention, values' clarification, behavior management, social and familial issues, and concerns specific to individual groups.

This chapter has addressed the consultation approach of training and education. This approach defined the consultant's role clarified as a consultant–trainer. The preparation for the training program was described with its stages of preplanning, contracting, topical development, arrangements to be made, and consultee participation. Concerns specific to the consultant inside an organization and a consultant outside an organization were addressed and differentiated. The implementation stage was described with emphasis on planning for and conducting the training session. The need for evaluations was presented as well as some directions for this part of the process. Issues of training conducted without follow-up consultation, ethical issues in training, and multicultural concerns in training were discussed. Finally, a checklist of concerns in accepting, organizing, and conducting the training program was provided.

REFERENCES

BARDON, J. (1985). On the verge of a breakthrough. *The Counseling Psychologist,* 13(3), 355–362.

BELLMAN, G. (1983). Untraining the trainer: Steps toward consulting. *Training and Development Journal,* January, 70–74.

CONOLEY, J. and CONOLEY, C. (1982). The effects of two conditions of client-centered consultation on student teacher problem descriptions and remedial plans. *Journal of School Psychology,* 20 (4), 323–328.

FISHER, L. (1986). Systems-based consultation with schools. In L. Wynne, S. McDaniel, and T. Weber (eds.), *Systems consultation: A new perspective for family therapy* (342–356). New York: The Guilford Press.

GALLESSICH, J. (1985). Toward a meta-theory of consultation. *The Counseling Psychologist,* 13 (3), 336–354.

GALLESSICH, J. (1982). *The profession and practice of consultation.* San Francisco: Jossey-Bass.

GIBBS, J. (1980). The interpersonal orientation in mental health consultation: toward a model of ethic variations in consultation. *Journal of Community Psychology,* 8, 195–207.

GIBBS, J. (1985). Can we continue to be color-blind and class-bound? *The Counseling Psychologist,* 13 (3), 426–435.

HANSEN, J. (1977). Prevention through teacher consultation. *The Journal of School Health,* May, 289–292.

HANSEN, J. and HIMES, B. (1977). Critical incidents in consultation. *Elementary School Guidance and Counseling,* 11 (4), 291–295.

HANSEN, J. and HIMES, B. (Unpublished). An interpersonal communication and behavior modification training program for parents. A paper based on consultation within the Niagara Falls Community Mental Health Center, Niagara Falls, New York.

IMBER-BLACK, E. (1986). The systemic consultant and human service provider systems. In L. Wynne, S. McDaniel, and T. Weber (eds.), *Systems consultation: A new perspective for family therapy* (357–373.) New York: The Guilford Press.

INOUYE, K., and PEDERSEN, P. (1985). Cultural and ethnic content of the 1977 to 1982 American Psychological Association convention programs. *The Counseling Psychologist,* 13 (4), 639–648.

KATZ, T. (1984). Hostile audience: Proceed with caution! *Training and Development Journal,* February, 78–83.

KNOFF, H. (1985). Discipline in the schools: An inservice and consultation program for educational staffs. *The School Counselor,* January, 211–218.

KURPIUS, D. (1985). Consultation interventions: Successes, failures and proposals. *The Counseling Psychologist,* 13 (3), 368–389.

STEIN, T. (1975). Some ethical considerations of short-term workshops in the principles and methods of behavior modification. *Journal of Applied Behavior Analysis,* 8, 113–115.

STEWART, K., and MEDWAY, F. (1978). School psychologists as consultants: Issues in training, practice, and accountability. *Professional Psychology,* November, 711–718.

WEBER, T., McDANIEL, S., and WYNNE, L. (1986). Signposts for a Systems Consultation. In L. Wynne, S. McDaniel, and T. Weber, (eds.), *Systems consultation: A new perspective for family therapy* (29–34). New York: The Guilford Press.

CHAPTER NINE
CONSULTATION
THROUGH
PROGRAM EVALUATION

Program evaluation is a form of applied research. That is, program evaluation is scientific investigation directed toward clinical and administrative concerns. Since these concerns are quite varied, program evaluation includes such diverse areas as agency accountability, cost-benefit analysis, needs assessment, management information systems, and outcome evaluations.

Program evaluation frequently involves outcome evaluations. Here the consultant is asked to design a research methodology that will accurately evaluate a program's effectiveness. The primary question is: Does the program work? Depending on the answer to this question, the consultant may also be asked to provide a description of the program's process (thereby explaining why the program does or does not work) as well as recommendations for change.

This chapter will begin with a review of the evaluation consultant's roles and functions. A five-step method for performing a program evaluation is presented along with explanations of problems that typically plague outcome evaluations. Issues in program evaluation, such as difficulty in measuring program objectives, will also be addressed.

MULTIPLE ROLES OF EVALUATION

Attkisson and Broskowski (1978) note that program evaluation grew in importance during the 1970s because of the need to control and contain costs. This approach emphasizes the accountability aspect of program evaluation. Costs may be higher than necessary because of an overlap among services provided by an agency; similarly, more resources may be needed because treating one problem of living for an individual may have no effect on other problems. Attkisson and Broskowski (1978) also suggest that program evaluation informs decision making and aids future planning. Program evaluators make reasonable judgments about programs based upon systematic data collection and analysis.

Program evaluators can provide information for communication outside and within the organization (Attkisson, Brown, and Hargreaves, 1978). Attkisson and colleagues (1978) also suggest that program evaluation can provide assistance with system resource management (clarifying objectives, planning, allocating resources, determining fees and billing rates), client utilization (assure access to service, quality assurance), intervention outcomes (detect ineffective services, determine cost-effectiveness), and community impact (regional health planning, integration of services with other agencies).

Barnes, Brook, Hesketh, and Johnson (1985) suggest that process evaluations, rather than outcome evaluations, may be more useful for service providers. Process evaluations systematically examine the inner workings of a program. Barnes and associates suggest that process evaluations can describe (1) what has been evaluated; (2) the theoretical basis of the intervention; (3) the skill level of the implementing staff; and (4) the characteristics of the target population.

PROGRAM EVALUATION STEP-BY-STEP

Attkisson and colleagues (1978) describe a five-step process which may be applied across program evaluation problems. Completion of all five steps in any evaluation is recommended. Examples are included to illustrate each step. A more thorough description of the difficulties common in program evaluation follows presentation of this method.

Identify the Specific Problem

Whether one is concerned with a needs assessment, process evaluation, or program evaluation, the problem to be studied must be specified as concretely as possible. The consultant should begin by asking the consultee to describe the problem to be studied. In some instances, the consultee may be able to describe the problem quite specifically. For example, an administrator may be interested in knowing which of two agencies are more successfully connecting clients with needed referral sources. To make matters simple, the consultee defines success as the client attending at least one meeting with the referral source.

On the other hand, the problem may be vague or multifaceted. In some cases, the consultee may be unable to describe precisely what constitutes success for these clients, and so it is left to the consultant to develop measures of success. For example, an administrator may wish to know which of two agencies employing different methods is more successful in providing effective vocational counseling to a group of unemployed high school dropouts. The consultant might start this process by reviewing the literature on outcome evaluation with vocational counseling programs and searching for applicable outcome measures. Such a review might produce an instrument like the Career Maturity Inventory (Crites, 1978), which assesses the extent to which clients are ready to pursue career exploration and decision tasks, or even such a simple task as asking clients to generate a list of acceptable vocational choices. Effective counseling would increase the number of potential vocations for persons who are beginning the exploration process.

Even when the problem definition task has been left to the consultant, it is wise to return to the consultee (and other important constituents) before the investigation starts and reach a consensus that the proposed measures represent information that the consultee desires. In general, the consultant should check with the consultee throughout the consultation process. If the consultant fails to do so, and the results of the study are undesirable, the consultee may be tempted to claim that the evaluation measured no meaningful variables and that recommended changes are worthless.

As Ziegenfuss and Lasky (1980) note, the problem identification stage is an opportunity to develop a relationship with the consultee. They conclude that literature reviews "suggest that the lack of success of evaluation appears more attitudinal than technological" (p. 666). Developing a relationship between evaluator and consultee may increase the chances that the agency eventually follows the consultant's recommendations.

Gather Relevant Information and Analyze

In this step, the consultant employs the problem definition to select the research design and statistical analyses. If a question arises about what services an agency should offer, a needs assessment would follow. If an agency desires to know why a particular program is functioning poorly, a process evaluation is a logical step. If information is needed about the effectiveness of a particular program, an outcome evaluation is performed.

With some exceptions, outcome evaluations involve the comparison of two or more groups. Exceptions involve evaluations of a single group. For example, an evaluator may administer a pretest, follow clients through an agency's intervention, and then administer a posttest. The evaluator analyzes the data by comparing posttest scores with pretest scores. However, even if a statistically significant change from pre- to posttest is found, doubt exists about whether the change resulted from the intervention or other factors.

If forced to employ only one group, evaluators can strengthen their confidence by replicating a previous study. In essence, the evaluator can find a previous study which employed a similar treatment and clients and run the evaluation as closely as possible to the previous study (for example, using the same measuring instruments). The evaluator may then compare the evaluation's results to previous findings. In the final analysis, however, the evaluator needs a control or comparison group to rule out alternate explanations. These issues are discussed in greater detail below under the heading Problems of Internal Validity.

Control groups are composed of individuals who do not receive the intervention but do complete the study's measures. For example, if a consultant is asked to assess the effectiveness of an agency's vocational counseling program, she or he may assign new clients to the counseling program or to a waiting-list control group. In the waiting-list control, clients wait until the treatment group is finished before they are assigned to treatment; during the study they complete the same instruments as the treatment group. Should the evaluator find changes in the vocational counseling group when compared to the control, our confidence increases that the change resulted from the treatment program.

That confidence, however, is also affected by *how* clients were assigned to the treatment or control group. If clients were randomly assigned, then we have more confidence that the individuals who began in the counseling and control groups were approximately equal. If random assignment was not employed, then we may have two different groups of clients. When the control and treatment groups differ on individual characteristics (such as gender or intelligence), we have no way of knowing whether differences that show up at posttest are a result of the intervention or individual characteristics. In the vocational counseling study described above, nonrandom assignment might result in most of the older students being placed in the counseling group. Examination of posttest scores might then show treatment clients to possess higher scores than controls on a measure of career maturity because of the age of the clients, not treatment effects.

Whether or not clients are randomly assigned, it is a good idea to have clients complete pretest measures to determine the equivalency of groups on study measures. If the groups differ, it is possible to control statistically for the differences by using the analysis of covariance statistical procedure.

Researchers use the term *quasi-experiment* to describe studies in which subjects are not randomly assigned to groups. As noted above, random assignment is preferable because it reduces the number of alternate explanations for the results of a study. Quasi-experiments, however, appear to be more frequently conducted in program evaluation. Administrators may set limits on time or fees which restrict the evaluator.

A school principal, for example, may wish to know whether a new AIDS education curriculum is effective with high school students. A program evaluator might compare a treatment group (a class which receives the AIDS education) with a control group (another class which receives no AIDS education) or a comparison group (another class which receives standard health and sex education). Because each group consisted of an existing class (i.e., no random assignment), this would be a quasi-experiment; the different composition of the classes might account for any differences found between them. Students could be pretested and posttested on measures assessing knowledge about AIDS, attitudes toward AIDS, and self-reported incidence of sexual behavior which carries a high risk of AIDS infection. If the comparison involved the AIDS-education and no-education classes, the consultant may very well find differences between the groups and recommend that the school implement AIDS education for all students. If the comparison involved the AIDS education and sex/health education classes, the consultant would probably find smaller differences between the groups. Costs of the new AIDS education class might be calculated and contrasted with the extent of improvement on students' AIDS knowledge, attitudes, and behavior.

Mitchell and Thompson (1985) discuss two measures of cost: (1) cost-effectiveness, which determines the relative costs for each intervention, and (2) cost-benefit, which determines the costs given the beneficial outcomes of different interventions. Direct and indirect costs can be included in cost analysis, such as the resources to deliver treatment or lost productivity. See Rossi, Freeman, and Wright (1979) for further discussion of cost-benefit procedures.

Evaluators who perform needs assessment may conduct surveys to obtain data, typically through telephone interviews or paper-and-pencil questionnaires. Dillman (1978) offers practical suggestions for questionnaire design that include (1) reduction of the survey to a small-sized booklet to increase respondents' perception that the survey is easy to do; (2) attention to the physical attractiveness of the booklet; (3) pretesting of the survey; (4) explanation in a cover letter that the survey is intended to be a vehicle to solve an important social issue; (5) follow-ups to the initial mailings; and (6) extensive personalization, such as including the respondent's name on the cover letter.

The quality of data available for a program evaluation is extremely variable. Agencies with excellent service programs may have funding difficulties because of administrative problems in record keeping (Ziegenfuss and Lasky, 1980). In such settings the evaluator may find it useful to develop an evaluation manual which directs the acquisition of information about administration, services, fiscal management, legal affairs, and clerical services. Data could be available in patient care records, personnel records, and logs. Using information routinely gathered at the evaluation site is preferred because the results of the evaluation will then be most readily understood. Assessments routinely employed in clinical and research settings are the next most desirable form because they offer a comparison based on normative data or evaluations at other sites. Finally, evaluators may elect to create instruments specific to the program evaluation. This last option is the least desirable because the evaluator may lack the resources necessary to gather reliability and validity data necessary to demonstrate the instrument's psychometric properties.

Attkisson and associates (1978) note that when trying to assess every client, economy is an important consideration. Many treatment evaluators simply take a measure of global functioning along with a rating of client satisfaction. An example of a rating system of global functioning is the Global Assessment of Functioning Scale (GAF; described on p. 12 of the *Diagnostic & Statistical Manual of Mental Disorders—Revised,* American Psychiatric Association, 1987), which enables the clinician to rate the client's problem severity on a 1 to 90 scale. A more detailed assessment, perhaps including an interview, might be carried out with a small sample.

Problems that plague assessment in clinical and research settings also appear in program evaluation (Atkisson et al., 1978; see Kazdin, 1980). Ratings may be biased: clients may want to appear "sick" so as to continue to receive benefits, while treatment providers may rate outcomes as overly positive because their positions may be affected by evaluation results. Global ratings may obscure specific changes, and long-range outcomes may be unrelated to short-term changes. In general, assess as many different outcomes, over as long a period of time, as is feasible. Multiple-outcome measures may offset some of the problems mentioned above and may be useful in post-hoc explanations.

Clients who partake in program evaluations also have a right to decline such participation. Informed consent typically includes information about alternative services available if clients choose not to participate, potential benefits and risks of the study, and any procedures required of participants that are not part of routine services. Clients should be able to terminate without penalty and be given the name and phone number of the investigator running the evaluation.

Generate Understandable Reports

Once the study and analyses have been completed, the consultant must find a way to communicate results and recommendations back to the consultee. If the consultant has consistently communicated with the consultee throughout the process, the report generation phase will be easier. A consensus should have been reached about problem definition and assessment; the consultant should have explained how the problem was being studied. This information should be presented in a written report that is tailored to the needs of the consultee.

The best way to write this tailored report is to ask the consultee what information should be communicated or emphasized. The consultee may possess different interests regarding the evaluation's sampling procedure, instrument selection, research methodology, statistical results, conclusions, and recommendations. Ask what the consultee wants and describe this information in language free of jargon and understandable to the consultee.

Propose and Review Alternatives

This step and the next depend upon the initial contract negotiated between consultee and consultant. Some consultees simply want the evaluator to provide information which they will employ to make decisions. On the other hand, the philosophy of Attkisson and associates (1978) is to involve the consultant throughout the process, including generation of alternatives and decision making. They believe that the consultant understands the program evaluation more thoroughly than anyone else and therefore should be present to make recommendations and decisions based on that evaluation. Attkisson et al. (1978) suggest that evaluators be part of decision making, particularly when "program managers lack skill in relating program information to decision options" (p. 83).

Implement the Decision with Continual Monitoring

Once the program evaluation is complete, there exists the very real possibility that no action will be taken. Consultants can avoid this by negotiating in the consultation contract that they will be present to help implement the decision and establish further monitoring. For example, if a particular method of vocational counseling is demonstrated to be superior, the consultant may explain the evaluation's results to counselors who will learn the new methods. The consultant may be able to make recommendations regarding training of the counselors.

In any event, the consultant should recommend that data gathering continue. Once an evaluation has been performed, it becomes easier to implement information gathering as part of an agency's regular routine. For example, the consultant may help establish a system of note-taking by counselors which briefly summarizes each client session. Supervisors might review these process notes to insure that the new counseling methods are being consistently applied. Similarly, every client who completes vocational counseling might complete all or part of the evaluation's outcome measures as a way to continue to monitor the quality of the program.

As an example of monitoring outcomes, Atkisson and colleagues (1978) report an evaluation designed to improve the acceptance rate of clients into a community mental health center. Initial evaluations indicated that relatively few clients were accepted per number of initial contacts. Debate within the agency followed, and a new, central intake unit was established. Data indicated that during the first month, 50 percent more clients were accepted. Additional monitoring through the next *three years* indicated that the intake unit continued to function adequately. It is again worth noting that once data collection procedures have been established in a program evaluation, it may be very worthwhile to leave those procedures in place as a method of monitoring programs and changes in programs.

PROBLEMS OF INTERNAL VALIDITY

With any type of research, one should be concerned with maximizing *internal* and *external* validity. Internal validity has to do with the veracity of the (usually causal) relationships one is investigating in a study. Thus, we might be concerned with whether a particular treatment approach really does decrease clients' depression. External validity has to do with how generalizable our study findings are. If we found that our treatment did decrease depression, we would then be concerned with whether the results would also apply to other clients, in other settings, working with other therapists who are employing our treatment approach.

Conflicts arise when one attempts to maximize *both* internal and external validity. When we focus upon internal validity, we are only interested in establishing a particular relationship (for example, treatment decreases depression). To do so, we must do everything possible to discount possible alternate explanations for our findings. Thus, in our depression treatment study, other explanations for our findings might include that therapists' expectations (and not the treatment per se) led to improvement or that our clients were already improving when they came into therapy and would have improved even without treatment. To be confident that our causal factor really operates, we want to eliminate such rival explanations. We might keep our therapists blind to the hypotheses of our study (thereby negating the influence of their expectations on clients) or we might include a no-treatment control group (to assess the degree of improvement that occurs without treatment). The problem, at least with more academically inclined research, is that we can become so concerned with questions of internal validity that we lose sight of external validity. Thus, we might so strongly control for possible alternate explanations in our study that our results cannot be generalized very easily to other settings. We may have set up so many special conditions (in terms of therapists, treatments, and clients) that our results are likely to be applicable only to this specific study.

Readers with research experience will understand that replication (repeating the study in a different time or setting) is crucial to establish external validity. In terms of program evaluation, however, there is often little concern about external validity. That is, when one conducts a needs assessment or an outcome evaluation, very often the persons who hire the consultant have no interest in knowing whether research conducted in their settings generalizes to other places. The only generalization they are concerned about is whether the results found in this program evaluation will generalize to the future in this agency and setting. Thus, in many cases in program evaluation, we can deemphasize concerns about external validity and focus primarily on internal validity.

Surprisingly, this is not often the case in actual program evaluation. The tone of many such investigations is extremely loose, and rival explanations abound. The major obstacle to rigorous research in program evaluation seems to be the organizational constraints with which evaluators must cope. The most important constraint is the inability to randomly assign clients (to treatment groups, for example) or to randomly select clients (for a needs assessment, for example).

An additional difficulty is the problem, discussed above, that many administrators have with understanding the research process. An evaluator may reason that since the person who hired them cannot or does not want to understand the nuances of the evaluation, no gain is made by paying close attention to internal validity considerations. Similarly, evaluators may lack the time or resources to perform what they perceive as additional work. Finally, evaluators may not want to know about possible confounds, partially because there may be nothing they can do about them.

Cook and Campbell (1979) describe a multitude of problems that can plague researchers in applied settings. The most important difficulties are described below.

Low Statistical Power

Evaluators who are interested in assessing differences among groups are likely to run into this difficulty. Sample size (the number of people in treatment groups, for example) and the size of the difference between groups on measuring instruments affect the sensitivity of statistical tests. Thus, larger samples and larger differences between groups are more likely to produce statistically significant results. In practical terms, this means that evaluators who assess groups with 20 or fewer persons per group will need substantial mean differences between groups for statistical tests to indicate that those differences are significant.

Reliability of Measures

Reliability refers to a measuring instrument's ability to consistently assess the variable it was designed to measure. Measures of low reliability cannot be depended upon to register true change. Thus, when you choose instruments for your evaluation, determine their reliability. This information is usually reported in manuals accompanying the assessments or in research reports describing their development. As a general guideline, reliability estimates should not be lower than .70.

Problems with low statistical power and low reliability of measures are possible in any study. Additional problems that particularly affect program evaluations occur when those evaluations examine groups in which the members have not been randomly assigned. As described above, random assignment refers to a procedure whereby every individual has an equal chance of being assigned to groups. Random assignment is the best method of insuring that the groups are approximately equal on all variables that might be influenced by treatment.

When groups are not randomly assigned, special problems arise. As noted above, these problems have to do with the possibility that any differences between groups have more to do with group composition than any intervention. Cook and Campbell's (1979) list of these potential threats to internal validity is described below.

History

History refers to the possibility that an event that occurs outside of the study might affect clients. For example, you are evaluating a stress reduction program at a local company. You have not been able to randomly assign clients to the stress reduction and control groups because management is interested only in reducing stress in the Research and Development department. As a quasi-control group, you selected the Marketing Department because of their similarity to R&D personnel in terms of age, experience, and pretest scores on a stress instrument, the Maslach Burnout Inventory.

Six weeks into your eight-week program the company is purchased in a hostile takeover. New management has announced that they intend to dissolve the R&D department in order to pay for the junk bonds that financed the takeover attempt. You complete your stress reduction program, administer the posttests to treatment and control groups, and discover that (1) the R&D mean scores of stress have doubled since the pretest and (2) the R&D mean scores are significantly higher than the Marketing Department's. Would you conclude that your stress reduction program had a paradoxical effect? Or might you consider the possibility that history played a role?

Maturation

Clients may change as a result of normal development (i.e., people naturally become older, wiser, etc.). It may become difficult to separate these maturation effects from treatment effects.

For example, as a consultant you may be asked to evaluate the effects of a university's freshman orientation program on social maturity. The university is interested in implementing a year-long program for freshman that would decrease students' problematic behavior such as alcohol and drug abuse or dropping out. Because of maturation, students would be expected to become more socially responsible as they go through their college education. Consequently, if the orientation program had no control or comparison group, it would be difficult to know whether changes in students' behavior, from their freshman to senior years, were a result of maturation or the intervention. Similarly, if the orientation program was run on a voluntary basis, you could compare a group of program volunteers and nonvolunteers on measures of social maturity. It may be, however, that volunteers were more mature to begin with or that they matured at a faster rate than the comparison group. Without random assignment to a control group, you would have a difficult time suggesting that changes in behavior resulted solely from the intervention and not from maturation.

Testing

Repeated administrations of a test can lead to effects that are unrelated to treatment. For example, familiarity with items might change clients' scores. With increased exposure, clients may decipher the aims of the scales and change their answers in a way that they expect would please the evaluator or make them look good. Similarly, repeated testing may help clients figure out the content of the test and help them improve their scores independent of new knowledge.

Instrumentation

How you measure variables influences the effects you find. For example, there may be changes in the measuring instrument between pretest and posttest.

Suppose you were interested in assessing whether social-skills training improved interpersonal interactions of a group of schizophrenics. You might have raters watch videotaped role plays of clients and rate them on such variables as eye contact, tone of voice, and overall effectiveness in communication. As they gain experience, the raters could conceivably be changing how they rate the tapes; for example, they might become more critical in their ratings of overall effectiveness over time. If this negative effect increased as raters assessed pre- and then posttest tapes, treatment gains may be offset by changes in instrumentation (i.e., the raters).

Statistical Regression

It is a common phenomenon that persons whose scores lie at the extremes of a group will tend to move back toward the mean upon retesting. This regression toward the mean is more pronounced with unreliable measures. Regression becomes problematic for program evaluators when they are examining research in which there are small numbers of subjects and when one or more of those subjects has extreme scores (particularly at pretest). Regression effects then make it more difficult to determine true differences between groups.

Selection

How are persons selected for treatment and control groups? This problem refers to differences in the kinds of people in one group versus another. Selection problems are characteristic of quasi-experiments because groups composed of *different* types of persons receive treatments. In contrast, randomized experiments are composed of groups whose members had equal probability of being assigned to them and who therefore are more likely to be equal on a large number of variables.

You might decide to evaluate a consultation project designed to increase physicians' abilities and willingness to assess patients' psychosocial problems. In this project physicians were self-selected, that is, they volunteered for your course about psychosocial problems. If you compared this group of physicians at the end of the course with physicians in the hospital who did not volunteer, you would be likely to find differences in their willingness to assess psychosocial problems. You would not know, however, if these differences were a result of your course or the self-selected physicians' motivation to learn. You might be able to partially rule out motivation as an alternate explanation by checking both groups' pretest scores on the willingness measure. If, however, even volunteer and nonvolunteer physician scores were equal at pretest, you still would not know if future differences were due to the course or motivation. Thus, volunteers might very well learn at a faster rate or forget less than nonvolunteers because of their motivation.

Mortality

Different kinds of persons may drop out of a treatment group, thereby changing the composition of the experimental group from pretest to posttest. This problem can affect randomized and quasi-experimental evaluations alike.

For example, suppose you are hired to assess the effects of a new alcohol treatment at a community mental health center. You begin with a pool of 40 subjects and randomly assign 20 to the treatment and 20 to a waiting-list control. At the end of your six-month treatment, however, only 10 persons remain in the treatment group. You compare treatment and control groups and find that the treatment group is significantly lower in alcohol consumption. Can you conclude that your treatment is effective? It may be that persons who dropped out did so because the treatment was ineffective or harmful (Hansen, Collins, Malotte, Anderson, Johnson, and Fielding, 1985). If these persons had completed posttreatment measures, differences between control and treatment groups might have been insignificant.

At the conclusion of any evaluation involving groups, determine the proportion of dropouts in each group. It's useful information in and of itself to know which, if any, groups produced the largest amount of attrition. If time allows, follow up on the dropouts to determine if they left because they received what they wanted, they felt they were getting worse, or they did not believe the treatment was effective.

Ceiling and Floor Effects

Ceiling and floor effects refer to the highest and lowest levels that an instrument can measure. With ceiling effects, the instrument cannot register any further gain; with floor effects, the instrument cannot demonstrate any further decrease.

For example, let us assume that you are assessing the effects of a stress reduction group with an instrument that has a possible range from 0 (no stress indicated) to 100 (very stressed). Unknown to you, the company where you are performing the stress reduction and evaluation had previously hired a consultant who taught meditation techniques to employees. It so happens that the employees who volunteer for your group have continued practicing the relaxation exercises. At pretest their mean scores on your instrument are 5.0 (indicating very little stress). They complete your treatment and at posttest their mean scores are 4.0. You calculate a statistical test to determine pre–post differences and find that none exists. Did your treatment fail to work? Or did the floor effect of your instrument fail to indicate further progress made during the stress reduction group?

Similar effects can occur at the other end of the scale. You might be asked to assess the effects of leadership training for a group of successful executives. These executives' pretest scores on a test of leadership might be so high that the scale may be unable to demonstrate improvements that occur as a result of training.

The best way to avoid ceiling and floor effects is to test the instrument, before the actual study, with a small group similar to the one that will be employed in the program evaluation. In this way you can determine if the scale can show increases or decreases as a result of treatment.

Diffusion of Treatments

Treatment and control groups do not always experience separate conditions. It may be that the treatment group communicates with the control, thereby diffusing treatment. For example, a school may institute a new alcohol education program for an eighth-grade class. Hired as an evaluator, you discover that the class does not differ from a similar control class on posttest measures of alcohol knowledge, attitudes, or drinking intentions. You also learn, however, that the treatment class attended physical education with the control students immediately after their alcohol education sessions and were observed to talk together about alcohol. It may be that the treatment group shared the alcohol education intervention with the controls, thereby negating any differences on study measures.

Compensatory Equalization of Treatment

If treatments are seen as valuable, administrators may be pressured to give controls equal treatment for political or ethical reasons. For example, you may be asked to evaluate a program in which a large city receives a block grant to improve teachers' salaries in an effort to improve education. Teachers in 30 of 60 schools subsequently receive $5,000 raises. Halfway through the school year (and your evaluation), however, administrators bow to union pressure and find money to give the remaining teachers a raise of $3,500 each. If students at all schools are equivalent in achievement tests at the end of the school year, will you conclude that higher teacher salaries had no effect on student performance?

Political and ethical issues can also influence whether clients can be randomly assigned to treatment. Cook and Campbell (1979) suggest that an administrator's apprehension about randomization is based upon: (1) differences in desirability of treatment; (2) the probability that individuals will learn of the differences; (3) whether organized constituencies will learn of differences; and (4) how much the constituency will feel affected by likely research outcomes. Thus, randomization is more likely to be approved where study conditions have equal desirability, individuals and constituencies are unlikely to learn of different conditions, and constituencies expect to be unaffected by research results.

Compensatory Rivalry by Respondents Receiving Less Desirable Treatments

In some instances, controls may see themselves as underdogs and try harder. This is likely when treatment and control groups are publicly announced and competition is thus generated.

Where ethical and practical, employ unobtrusive measurements (see Webb, Campbell, Schwartz, Sechrest, and Grove, 1981). In addition to preventing competition, unobtrusive measures are less likely to generate reactivity in subjects. Unobtrusive measures are those methods of collecting data in which research subjects are unaware that they are being observed. For example, class attendance could be an unobtrusive measure if students did not know that their attendance was part of data collection. Subjects who are unaware of an evaluation's purpose and instruments may be more likely to respond in an unbiased manner. Similarly, a general orientation to a study—as compared to instructions which list the study's hypothesis and aim—is less likely to generate reactivity in subjects.

ASSESSMENT DEVELOPMENT AND EVALUATION

Evaluators need a basic knowledge of assessment both for selecting appropriate measures and for developing their own scales. As noted above, use of an existing measure is preferred because at least some data about the scale's properties are usually available. In terms of time and effort, it is always worth doing a literature search for appropriate instruments before investing the resources necessary to produce a psychometrically sound scale. Useful resources include Buros's Mental Measurements Yearbook, publications by the Test Corporation of America, or products like the Instrumentation Kit (University Associates, Inc., 8517 Productive Avenue, San Diego, Calif., 92121).

Nevertheless, evaluators may find they must develop a special scale for a particular evaluation. Dawis (1987) provides several guidelines regarding scale development. The best starting point is a theory of the construct that the scale is supposed to measure. This theory may aid in item creation by providing a specific definition of the variable, describing what it is and is not, and how it depends on and relates to other variables. It may also be useful to conduct open-ended interviews with clients at the evaluation site to gather content for items.

Scale developers must also select a response format such as true–false, multiple choice, or Likert. Dawis (1987) suggests four guidelines: (1) choose the simpler format; (2) more scale points are better than fewer; (3) use an even number of scale points to eliminate neutral responding; and (4) avoid ranking formats. These guidelines are designed to make the scales easy for respondents to understand and provide data that is most easily subjected to statistical analysis.

Dawis (1987) also suggests a small study to determine such practical considerations as how easily instructions were followed, how long it took to complete, and how appropriate the content appeared to respondents. Preliminary analyses could include calculation of a Cronbach *alpha* to determine the scale's internal consistency; computer programs like SPSS which calculate *alpha* usually provide options to examine item-total correlations. Deletion of items with low item-total correlations will increase scale reliability and validity. Also examine the range of response for each item; in general, items for which there is little variability (e.g., everyone answers "True") should be deleted because they fail to differentiate among respondents. Scales which demonstrate substantial variability among respondents are useful because they allow the researcher to differentiate among subjects on the construct in question.

Existing and developed scales may be evaluated by their reliability and validity estimates. Reliability refers to the consistency of measurement; the lower the reliability of a scale, the greater the amount of error or unknown influences. Validity refers to whether a scale measures what it is intended to measure; scales with low validity, for example, may be fairly useless in predicting outcomes of interest in a program evaluation.

More information about evaluating and developing scales may be obtained through reading such references as Crocker and Algina (1986), Ghiselli, Campbell, and Zedeck (1981), or Kaufman and Thomas (1980).

ISSUES

Attkisson and Broskowski (1978) note that many human service personnel see evaluation as an externally imposed requirement used to terminate unwanted programs or justify administrative decisions. They suggest, however, that the goal of evaluation is to improve programs and that multiple perspectives, including those of staff, clients, and administrators, exist about what constitutes improvement. Persons whose work is being evaluated, be they teachers, managers, or counselors, are often asked or required to spend considerable amount of time in recordkeeping for program evaluation purposes. Unfortunately, this information is seldom reported to these persons, much less in a timely manner that could influence their activities.

Attkisson and colleagues (1978) assert that "the complexities and difficulties of doing evaluation in applied settings are so great that the results of many such efforts have reduced credibility" (p. 61). Problems such as translating broad goals into measurable objectives, unstandardized delivery programs, and community hostility toward evaluation may all make the results of an evaluation difficult to interpret or invalid. Attkisson and colleagues also note that even when findings are valid, they may be irrelevant. For example, the outcome measures selected by investigators may not assess content that concerns administrators, or administrators may be unable to understand the complex data analyses.

The persons who design program evaluations are likely to be research- and statistically oriented; the products of research, whether intended for program evaluation or pure science, seldom are black-and-white, unconditional statements. At the same time, the administrators and executives who fund program evaluation often want relatively simple answers: Does a program accomplish its intended purpose or not? Consultees may have little interest in understanding the nuances of research and how they may affect the interpretation of program evaluations.

Ziegenfuss and Lasky (1980) cite Angrist (1975) as indicating that program evaluation can be stifled by "the urge for quick answers, the pressure to make informed decisions, and the danger that program monies and interest will wane . . . " (p. 666). A rigorous program evaluation may identify problems but fail to develop tools for implementing needed change. Carter (1971) suggests that most administrators equate program evaluation with program justification. Consultees may reject results which do not fit beliefs or needs. Negative results (i.e., that programs do not work) may be ignored outright.

Atkisson et al. (1978) also note that program evaluation results may be underutilized because managers are unable or unwilling to use the results. Similarly, change in programs is more likely to result from political factors (within and external to the organization) than from the simple feedback of a program evaluation. Evaluation may be a threat to the roles of the parties being evaluated (Barnes et al., 1985).

Program evaluators deal with organizational politics in different ways. Barnes and associates (1985) leaked the results of the evaluation before the final report was present. They assumed that by sharing the results early, key decision makers would have time to adjust to the report. Barnes et al.

also report being prepared for criticisms. They expected criticisms and listened openly and nondefensively. They also avoided criticizing any particular personnel and focused on program inputs in relation to goals in an effort to make discrepancies obvious. McCormack and DeVore (1986) reported that they contracted to distribute written reports of their evaluation to staff members and "prepared to decline the invitation to consult if a satisfactory feedback mechanism had not been agreed to" (p. 56).

Weiss (1983) listed criticisms of program evaluation in education which are applicable to other settings as well. Program evaluation is often too narrow in that evaluators may choose to assess variables that are relatively easy to measure (e.g., grade point average) as compared to variables that are important to the persons who are involved with the program (e.g., value development) or processes that could help program operators improve the program (e.g., why students drop out). Evaluation measures may be unrealistic in that they may set too high a standard for the program to meet (e.g., using reading scores as an outcome measure for a reading program that meets two times a week). Finally, program evaluation results are infrequently shared with staff and clients and often fail to influence decisions about the program.

SUMMARY

In this chapter a recommendation was made for rigorous program evaluation that emphasizes the elimination of alternate explanation of evaluation results. Such rigor, however, requires that consultants negotiate the resources and conditions for the evaluation before work begins. For example, consultants would be wise to educate administrators, clinicians, and clients about the desirability of randomly assigning subjects to treatment conditions.

In addition to evaluating program outcomes, consultants may provide a variety of services, including the development of management information systems as well as the selection and evaluation of mental health assessment instruments. Consultants should pursue these opportunities, however, with an awareness of the potential conflict engendered by the different perspectives of administrators, clinicians, clients, and evaluators.

REFERENCES

AMERICAN PSYCHIATRIC ASSOCIATION. (1987). *Diagnostic and statistical manual of mental disorders—revised (3rd ed.).* Washington, DC: Author.

ATTKISSON, C. C., BROWN, T. R., and HARGREAVES, W. A. (1978). *Roles and functions of evaluation in human service programs.* In C. C. Attkisson, W. A. Hargreaves, and M. J. Horowitz (eds.), *Evaluation of human service programs.* New York: Academic Press.

ATTKISSON, C. C., and BROSKOWSKI, A. (1978). Evaluation and the emerging human service concept. In C. C. Attkisson, W. A. Hargreaves, and M. J. Horowitz (eds.), *Evaluation of human service programs*. New York: Academic Press.

BARNES, J., BROOK, J., HESKETH, B., and JOHNSON, M. (1985). The professional psychologist as evaluator in a community agency setting. *Professional Psychology: Research & Practice*, 16, 681–688.

COOK, T. D., and CAMPBELL, D. T. (1979). *Quasi-experimentation*. Chicago: Rand McNally College Publishing Co.

CRITES, J. O. (1978). *Theory and research handbook for the Career Maturity Inventory*. Monterey, CA: California Test Bureau/McGraw-Hill.

CROCKER, L., and ALGINA, J. (1986). *Introduction to classical and modern test theory*. New York: Holt, Rinehart and Winston.

CZANDER, W. M. (1986). *The application of social systems thinking to organizational consulting*. New York: University Press of America.

DAWIS, R. V. (1987). Scale construction. *Journal of Counseling Psychology*, 34, 481–489.

DEMONE, H. W., SCHULBERG, H.C., and BROSKOWSKI, A. (1978). *Evaluation in the context of developments in human services*. In C. C. Attkisson, W. A. Hargreaves, and M. J. Horowitz (eds.), *Evaluation of human service programs*. New York: Academic Press.

DILLMAN, D. (1978). *The total design method*. New York: John Wiley.

GHISELLI, E. E., CAMPBELL, J. P., and ZEDECK, S. (1981). *Measurement theory for the behavioral sciences*. San Francisco: W. H. Freeman.

GREINER, L. E., and METZGER, R. O. (1983). *Consulting to management*. Englewood Cliffs, NJ: Prentice Hall.

HANSEN, W., COLLINS, L., MALLOTTE, C. K., ANDERSON JOHNSON, C., and FIELDING, J. (1985). Attrition in prevention research. *Journal of Behavioral Medicine*, 8, 261–275.

HARGREAVES, W. A., and ATTKISSON, C. C. (1978). *Evaluating program outcomes*. In C. C. Attkisson, W. A. Hargreaves, and M. J. Horowitz (eds.), *Evaluation of human service programs*. New York: Academic Press.

KAUFMAN, R., and THOMAS, S. (1980). *Evaluation without fear*. New York: New Viewpoints.

KAZDIN, A. (1980). *Research design in clinical psychology*. New York: Harper & Row.

McCORMACK, J., and DeVORE, J. (1986). Survey-guided process consultation in a veterans administration medical center psychology service. *Professional Psychology: Research and Practice*, 17, 51–57.

Mitchell, W.D., and Thompson, T.L. (1985). Some methodological issues in consultation-liaison psychiatry research. *General Hospital Psychiatry*, 7, 66–72.

SCHLESINGER, H., MUMFORD, E., GLASS, G., et al. (1983). Mental health treatment and medical care utilization in a fee-for-service system: Outpatient mental health treatment following the onset of a chronic disease. *American Journal of Public Health*, 73, 422–429.

ROSSI, P. H., FREEMAN, H. E., and WRIGHT, S. R. (1979). *Evaluation: A systematic approach*. Beverly Hills, CA: Sage.

WEBB, E., CAMPBELL, D., SCHWARTZ, R., SECHREST, L., and GROVE, J. (1981). *Nonreactive measure in the social sciences*. Boston: Houghton Mifflin.

WEISS, C. H. (1983). The stakeholder approach to evaluation: Origins and promise. In A. S. Bryk (ed.), *Stakeholder-based evaluation*. San Francisco: Jossey-Bass.

ZIEGENFUSS, J. T., and LASKY, D. I. (1980). Evaluation and organizational development: A management-consulting approach. *Evaluation Review*, 4 (5), 665–676.

CHAPTER TEN
MANAGING CONFLICT: THIRD-PARTY RESOLUTION

Conflict occurs almost everywhere, at home, school, work, in the neighborhood, in society, and between countries. A number of methods have been explored to manage conflict including avoidance, regulation, and resolution. Several methods of conflict resolution involve the intervention of a third-party as in mediation, arbitration, and conciliation. These methods have been used to resolve conflicts between individuals, groups, and larger organizations. Another type of third-party intervention that has gained acceptance is called third-party consultation.

Third-party consultation focuses on the consultants diagnosing and helping the disputing parties to understand and constructively resolve their conflict. This approach is noncoercive, nonevaluative, and focuses on exploration and problem solving in terms of the basic relationships rather than on settlement of specific issues. Third-party consultation differs from more traditional types of intervention in terms of the degree of coercion applied to the two parties, the flexibility of the interaction, and the nature of the objective (Fisher, 1972).

To explore the concepts and methods of third-party intervention, this chapter begins by focusing on the concepts of conflict behavior. This will provide a base of knowledge about the problems to be resolved and why certain methods of intervention may be used. A brief review of the traditional third-party interventions is presented prior to concentrating on third-party consultation. The later sections examine the intervention strategies used in consultation.

Most of the literature in conflict resolution by third-parties relate to industry. Although much of the material in this chapter will draw on those resources, the concepts are applicable to all interpersonal conflicts. One of the reasons for the increased use of third-party consultation has been the need for such strategies in informal as well as formal settings.

CONCEPTS OF CONFLICT

A perspective on interpersonal and intergroup conflict is necessary in establishing methods of managing or resolving a conflict. Blake, Shepard, and Mouton (1964) presented a model describing intergroup conflict in industry. The concepts are still appropriate and are applicable to most other settings as well. Although the focus is on intergroup conflict behavior, the similarity to interpersonal conflicts is apparent. The basic assumptions about conflict and the ideas of the need for interdependence affect how disputing people behave and how the consultant can intervene.

Blake, Shepard, and Mouton (1964) wrote a book for managers which focused on intergroup conflict and its management. The emphasis in this book is to understand the dynamics of conflict in industry and the methods of resolving such conflict. They believe knowledge of intergroup conflict can be used to derive useful guidelines for managers and others who have intergroup conflicts to resolve. The book's blending of behavioral information and guidelines in conflict management are very helpful for consultants.

Perspective

The behavior of two individuals in a business or industrial relation is determined by three or more forces: (1) the formal job description, which outlines the responsibility each person brings to the job situation; (2) their backgrounds of training and experience in both the business field and the specific corporation; (3) their behavior, which is influenced by the role each believes he/she fills as a representative of the particular group in the organization.

When people speak from the framework of their own job responsibilities they speak only for themselves. The disagreement between individuals, then, is a personal matter. Conflicts may occur, however, between individuals which are affected by their job descriptions. When an employee disagrees with a supervisor about a job-related issue, the procedure for resolving the conflict and the ultimate decision usually lie with the supervisor. The supervisor may resolve the situation him or herself, turn it over to a subordinate, make no decision, or may seek a third person to which both parties can agree. When two peer employees have a disagreement and are unable to resolve their differences, they can submit the decision to a common supervisor who can make a decision through this higher authority. When individuals are behaving for themselves or within their job responsibilities, they are often able to resolve their own differences or through a supervisory action.

The complexity of a conflict increases considerably when the disagreeing individuals represent different groups. Individuals generally are seen as representative of their group whenever they interact with different groups who are in some way interdependent. Organizations are generally composed of many small groups which are interdependent. As a representative, a group member's opinions and attitudes are influenced by the goals and norms that he shares with his own group. Norms of behavior and the expectations of his group members do not allow him to behave independently of the group's interest when disagreements arise between the two groups. The result is often that organizational needs for interdependence and cooperation among the groups are not met as well as required.

Basic Assumptions About Intergroup Disagreement

Blake, Shepard, and Mouton (1964) suggested that organizational staff must focus not only on effective methods of resolving intergroup disagreements but also on the dysfunctional methods which lead to undesirable, disruptive side effects. They describe some of the dysfunctional methods of resolving conflicts which need to be understood to avoid their repetition. Three basic assumptions and attitudes toward disagreement and its management are identified. The first basic assumption is that disagreement is inevitable and permanent. The assumption is that the disagreement between two people or groups must be resolved in favor of one or the other. This assumption holds that there is no other alternative. If the two positions are seen as mutually exclusive and neither side is willing to capitulate, then any of three possible resolutions may be used: (1) A win/lose power struggle may ensue to the point of capitulation by one side. (2) Resolution may be established through a third-party decision. (3) An agreement may be made not to determine an outcome, therefore leaving it to the arbitration of fate.

A second assumption is that conflict can be avoided since interdependence between the two sides is unnecessary. When conflict occurs between two sides they can dissolve it by reducing the interdependence in one of three ways: (1) One side can withdraw from the situation. (2) They can maintain or substitute indifference in attitude when there appears a conflict of interest. (3) The two sides may isolate themselves or be isolated from each other. Each of these three resolutions focuses on maintaining independence rather than attempting to achieve resolution and interdependence.

A third assumption is that agreement is possible in that means of resolving it need to be found, thereby maintaining interdependence. Effort need not be devoted to determining who is right and wrong, nor to either yielding something or gaining something. Rather an effort is made to discover a new resolution of the points of difference.

MANAGING CONFLICT

Each of these assumptions about conflict is related to a specific approach to managing disagreement. Blake, Shepherd, and Mouton (1964) describe the resolution behaviors on a continuum from a passive attitude to an active orientation. For example, when the people involved believe that conflict is inevitable and agreement is impossible, there are three possible resolutions or management of the conflict. One is to be very passive, leaving whatever happens to fate. At the active end of the continuum is a power struggle to determine who is going to win and who is going to lose. In the middle of that continuum is management left to third-party judgment, in which someone of a higher authority or an objective judge makes the decision.

In a situation where people believe the conflict is not inevitable yet an agreement is not possible, the passive position is one of indifference or ignoring the area of conflict. A more active position is one of withdrawing from the other side, while the middle ground is one of just working in isolation rather than through interdependence.

Finally, when the people believe there is a conflict but agreement is possible, the passive-management approach is one of peaceful coexistence, in other words, sort of smoothing over the differences so they can get along. The active-management point of view involves problem solving from both sides, each trying to work out a resolution. The moderate position would be to split the differences, to work out a compromise position or bargain the differences between the two sides.

An examination of each of these assumptions as it relates to achieving resolution between conflicting sides will clarify participant behaviors and possible third-party roles. Behaviors when parties believe conflict is inevitable will naturally differ from when they believe it is not inevitable or that agreement is possible.

Conflict Is Inevitable and Agreement Impossible

In a win/lose orientation to conflict, the two sides see their interests as mutually exclusive and no compromise is possible. The success of one side depends on the failure of the other. The actions and reactions of the two sides often deepen antagonism and destroy avenues of resolution rather than contributing to intergroup problem solving (Blake, Shepherd, and Mouton, 1964). Since consultants often work with people or programs where this orientation is exhibited, they will benefit from understanding these power struggles in order to constructively deal with them.

A series of experiments were conducted under artificially established conditions. The experimental situations, however, were psychologically real for the individuals participating. The controlled situations highlighted and provided measurement of a number of psychological and social aspects in a win/lose conflict, and the generalizations from these studies provide some insight into conflict management. Approximately 1,000 subjects participated in these studies in more than 150 almost-identical groups. Competitive situations were established so that there existed no realistic possibility for avoiding confrontation. First, intragroup and then intergroup situations were studied. Later, effective and ineffective conditions for reducing competitive tensions and conflict were identified and evaluated.

Dynamics of win/lose power struggles.   Blake and associates (1964) summarized the generalizations from these experiments and then the steps derived from them, which can lead to more healthy intergroup problem solving.

Under competitive circumstances, cohesion within a group increases. When adversaries approach, members close ranks to defend or attack. Former disagreements within a group tend to be put aside and they pull together for the common goal. Group tension is apparent. Disputes among members—which could be used for creative thinking and can lead to enrichment of the initial group position—tend to get snuffed out. There is group pressure for each individual to conform once the group has reached a certain point of entrenchment.

Prior to competitive conflict, power relations tend to be loose and poorly developed. Most members do not feel responsibility for their group's performance; however, when clear and sharp competitive positions are established, the stakes are higher. Individual personal pride and reputation merge with the group's reputation, and typically a pecking order among group members is established. Individuals may become leaders due to superior logic or expression or because of a stronger motivation to win. The members who may be less aggressive or more dependent may become followers. Sometimes they show satisfaction in their agreement while at other times they take little active part, possibly to hide their disagreement or concern for defeat. If those in the leadership structure fail to recognize the rights of others, internal strife may occur, though possibly not until after the intergroup conflict is resolved. Barriers for future intragroup cooperation may have been established.

Each group establishes a statement of its position. Once this position is created, the group is able to compare what they have stated to the contending group's perspective. However, win/lose conflicts tend to distort judgments, and members judge their own position superior as to the other's, losing their objectivity about both positions. With heightened disagreement and decreasing objectivity the two sides have difficulty with problem solving.

After examining the two different positions, groups tend to interact through representatives who will determine the winner and loser. There may be a public debate between representatives to clarify their similarities and differences. Rather than reducing the conflict and increasing objectivity these discussions tend to intensify the conflict. Subjectivity is promoted when there are competitive and mutually frustrating experiences between the two groups. There tends to be strong stereotype formations. Members of each group develop negative attitudes and these expressions in turn tend to accelerate the other side.

Groups tend to select a representative who is seen as strong due to personal domination in the group, ability to resist conforming pressures, and ability to face up to the problems rather than running away from them. As individuals these representatives are typically seen quite objectively by the members of both groups before they enter the conflict. As the conflict precedes, however, the reaction soon destroys that initial perception.

The conclusion from these studies has been that competition affects people's capacity to think, to understand, and to comprehend (Blake et al., 1964). In the research studies on win/lose conflict, each group studied the other's position until all members indicated that they had achieved an intellectual understanding of their adversary's position. Then an objective test covering the positions of the two groups was used. The results showed that win/lose attitudes did contaminate objective thinking. Such attitudes tended to minimize the commonalities between their two positions and focused on highlighting differences. People saw items as unique to their own side even when they were present on both sides. People also tended to recognize points in the other group's position more readily than recognizing points of agreement in both positions. Distortions were present, however, in that people identified points distinctive to their own position more accurately than they did the items which were distinctive only to the adversary position. It appears that the blind spots in intellectual understanding of the other position are not just due to one's familiarity with one's own group. Differences in understanding are influenced according to group membership, feelings of personal ownership, group identification, and defensiveness under the threat of defeat.

Resolution of differences.   When representatives meet to determine a winner and loser, each must remain loyal to the group perspective. A representative who functions impartially and takes an objective view is in danger of losing for the group since she/he might have to admit that the competitor's position is better than her/his own. Therefore, loyalty to the group establishes pressure that may overwhelm logic. Subjectively, the representative feels that he/she is acting on intellectual convictions and logic and that loyalty to the point of view is not the major factor. The urge to win frequently becomes paramount, and intellectual objectivity disappears. The studies on conflict resolution indicate that deadlock is the most frequent result from such representative negotiation.

The experiments also permitted the study of resolution through a third-party arrangement in which an impartial judge was used to produce a verdict. The judge examines and evaluates each group's position against preestablished criteria. Based on his/her evaluation one group is judged a winner, and thus the other a loser. He/she explains the criteria of evaluating both positions and presents the decision.

Impact of victory and defeat.   Members in winning groups congratulate one another, especially those who led the fight to victory. The positions of leadership are strengthened and those who follow them tend to become even more dependent on the winning leaders in the future. Within the losing groups, infighting and splintering occur, resulting in factions as members are critical of the people who led them astray. Discontent becomes apparent, and the doubts of less vocal members now are presented. The common result is a shift in the leadership pecking order with those who previously were lower in status moving up the pecking order. The replaced leaders may fight back to justify their actions and remain influential.

The group mentality in winning and losing groups is dramatically different. This is seen in terms of their reactions to the judge, the representatives, and also in the atmosphere of the groups. The members of the winning group feel the glow of victory and a dominant sense of complacency from success. It does not occur to them to examine their efforts and to look for better ways of working. Rather, they tend to let down and enjoy the fruits of success. The defeated group tends to become focused on figuring out the falacies of the operation that led to failure and assigning responsibilities for them.

Using third-party judgment in resolutions.   In a situation where two sides are locked in disagreement, there is a need to establish some means for bringing about a victory. When a deadlock is reached but both groups feel resolution is necessary, they may be willing to take a chance on victory or defeat through employing some mechanism to obtain a clear resolution. Often this is a third-party judgment. A third-party resolution may be used when the two groups have reached an impasse and believe that further interaction will not resolve the differences. The two sides do not anticipate that a neutral judgment will provide a path for mutual agreement; they only hope this will put an end to their immediate struggle. It is necessary to recognize that one of the parties may have to shift its mode of operation as a result of the ruling; they may have to change enough to bring their behavior in line with the ruling. Therefore, victory for one and defeat for the other are essentially inevitable.

When negotiations between the groups' representatives have ended in a deadlock, an arbitrator may be brought in to make a decision. In this new environment the two representatives are now in a powerless situation. The arbitrator has the power to reach a decision, and the two groups have relinquished all power over the outcome. All legal systems right up to the Supreme Court, are based on achieving resolutions through the use of a neutral third party. Because the arbitrator is outside of the two groups, both sides are expected to accept the outcome as impartial.

Once an arbitrator renders a decision, the group whose position is favored sees the arbitrator as being fair and unbiased because the judgment proves that they were right in the first place. To those in the losing group the resolution retains an arbitrary and mechanical quality. They comply because the ground rules require it, but they remain unconvinced. In studies of intergroup competition, the immediate response of losing group members was to remain confident that their position is correct and that the arbitrator has been wrong; however, a delayed reaction among the members was that it is the group who is at fault. This reaction usually arises from members who were least committed to the group's position before it was submitted to arbitration or by those who prized their membership highest. In industrial arbitration, once the third-party judge renders a decision there is a likelihood that the group who wins will feel the uplift of victory and the losing group the pain of defeat. Therefore, a third-party judgment usually does not diminish the group's convictions about the win/lose nature of their disagreement.

Third-party arbitrators vary greatly in their approach to the arbitration. Some judgments are considered particularly effective when neither group feels like winners. The judge can assume a role of a mediator, counselor, or third-party intervener to bring about better understanding and mutual respect and enhance the ability of both sides to come to agreements in the future.

When a manager or supervisor serves as the third-party judge within his or her own organization, it may lead to further complications. Leaders of certain groups in an organization may turn to, or may be required to submit to, a common supervisor for the resolution of differences. When a supervisor or manager hears the two sides and makes a decision, that decision is made with primary consideration for the welfare of the organization. However, when acting as a third-party judge in an organization, a manager can create victories and losses among those between whom unity of effort is most needed. If a manager believes competition between groups for whom he or she is responsible is good for the organization, he or she can produce conditions that lead to subordinate groups viewing their differences as inevitable, possibly leading to further win/lose competitive situations and all the psychological struggles involved. In addition to open win/lose decisions which supervisors must decide, there are hidden win/lose conflicts that occur in the "back alleys" of the organization. The internal politics of an organization may involve efforts on the part of some individuals to try to gain sympathy for the correctness of their point of view.

Fate as a resolution.   When two groups are in conflict and disagreement is considered inevitable but a resolution is compelling, the use of fate in a decision is a third alternative. When people are involved in a win/lose power struggle but the direct confrontation by one group has not succeeded over the other, or through the action of a third-party judge, in the absence of an acceptable arbitrator to both sides the groups may turn to a purely mechanical technique of decision making. Flipping a coin is the classical example. It is interesting to note that intelligence is not used but rather mechanisms of chance become preferred as a basis for relieving the disagreement.

It is possible to combine a third-party judge with fate in the resolution decision. For example, an arbitrator is called upon to make a decision between two alternatives; when equal evidence is found on both sides, he or she may deliberate privately and essentially flip a coin before making a public decision. If the truth of this process becomes known to the two groups, it may well generate problematic reactions. The victory is taken away from one group, but defeat is not taken away from the other. Actually, there would then be two losers, and both groups would have negative attitudes toward the judge who had tricked them. Hidden decisions, based on fate, may generate even greater problems when the truth is discovered (Blake et al., 1964).

More common than tossing a coin but still a form of relying on fate is the behavior of procrastination. When group leaders delay or put off confrontation of an issue in the hopes that the problem will go away or that some new circumstance will resolve the issue, this handling of unresolved conflict is really a strategy of avoidance or denial, leaving resolution up to fate. When supervisors or managers in an organization are not sure which decision to make, they too may also postpone action. Essentially, they are using the mechanism of fate and hoping that something will happen on the job to remove them from responsibility for the decision.

Pure fate resolutions such as flipping a coin or drawing straws are seldom used in resolving major conflicts; however, some character of chance is often found in the way individuals or groups resolve their differences. In certain situations, fate-decision may seem the only answer. However, resorting to such a procedure may unwittingly result in even greater problems than were initially found in the disagreement.

Conflict Not Inevitable, Agreement Not Possible

One of Blake and associates (1964) basic assumptions about intergroup disagreement and their conflict management occurs when the members believe that conflict is not inevitable yet agreement is impossible. In these situations conflict management or resolution is accomplished by withdrawal, isolation, or indifference. These conditions are not based on an interdependence of these groups but on maintaining independence of their activities. Disagreement between these groups is not always inevitable as in a win/lose orientation, but neither is agreement seen to be possible. Therefore, they seek to withdraw from each other, function in isolation, or live with indifference toward the other position. Individuals and groups with this assumption do not seek a third party for resolution and resist when encouraged to use it.

Indifference and ignorance.   Members of a group may be interdependent with another group yet fail to see the logic of their interdependence. They may see no reason for any arrangement other than separation. Failure to see an interdependence is often found in organizations. Groups in a decentralized organization often, through ignorance, duplicate each other's efforts without being aware of it. At other times the duplication exists in a competitive sense—a refusal to understand the interdependence and how it could improve their work.

Indifference or a position of neutrality may occur when a group abandons attempts to cooperate or avoids competitive contact with another group. Contact and communication with the other group are reduced and sometimes entirely eliminated. The problems that exist between the groups may be the reason why the group cannot achieve its purpose. Ignorance and indifference are considered passive methods of resolving a problem.

Isolation. A middle ground between passive indifference and active withdrawal is isolation behavior. Contact is reduced and walls are erected which make interdependence unnecessary. In such a situation each group can proceed according to its own description of the problem without needing to respond to the influence of the other group.

Isolation is most frequently found in organizations with a decentralized administration. Decentralization proceeds with the notion that administrators who are delegated authority to build their division will nevertheless be aware of their interdependence with the rest of the organization. A frequent weakness in decentralization, however, is managers' failure to recognize that interdependence. The disadvantages of isolation as a method of reducing or avoiding conflict are numerous. The most important involves the loss of interchange which could be mutually stimulating and profitable for both parties. There is also long-term loss for the organization. When groups cannot agree, they often try to work in isolation. Where they perceive that disagreement is inevitable, they may split, each going their own way. The potential advantages of interdependence and seeking the best solution are thereby lost.

Withdrawal. Groups or individuals who have experienced repeated victory or defeat from win/lose struggles may withdraw from the larger organization. A particularly successful group may develop an attitude of superiority and a type of isolation. The attitude toward other groups or organizations becomes that they are not needed and the successful group does not want to become dependent on others. Attitudes and behaviors consistent with withdrawal are more common of groups or individuals who have suffered numerous defeats. They may try to limit contacts with other groups or members in other groups to those which are required by the work situation. The internal reactions of such a group are to realign its power structure, and frequently the authority structure limits the freedom of its members, the group leader becoming the primary contact person with outside groups.

Withdrawal attitudes and behaviors are also characterized by absence of initiative. Such groups view themselves as providing services rather than initiating new ideas. There may be a sense of threat in this group. Other groups with similar functions are avoided, being seen as competitors rather than as offering opportunities for collaboration. A group in withdrawal may also experience subgrouping into mutual disparaging cliques. Clearly, the separation reduces contact with other individuals or groups with whom interdependence exists and thereby reduces the need to achieve agreement in new areas.

Although There Is Conflict, Agreement Is Possible

Another category in intergroup relations is concerned with groups that assume that although disagreement is present, agreement is possible. There are three levels of activity for groups in achieving intergroup cooperation: Peaceful coexistence is the most passive condition. Compromise mechanisms represent a more active approach to working together. And problem solving is the most active.

Peaceful coexistence.   Under the condition of peaceful coexistence, groups tend to exercise their commonalities and play down differences. Group goals and norms of behavior which might conflict with those of another tend to be isolated, either by an implicit or explicit agreement between the groups. An attitude of tolerance is the norm of conduct for areas of disagreement. To operate effectively in a large organization numerous decisions are made, implying that there will be many differing points of view that need to be resolved. If the organization has little or no intergroup conflict, it is likely that a state of peaceful coexistence has been achieved. Groups try to avoid issues that would divide them, and different points of view that might generate a win/lose struggle are not discussed. In hierarchical positions in organizations, subordinates tend to feel powerless and tend to direct their energies toward coexistence and harmony. Similarly, peer groups often feel compelled to follow a position of peaceful coexistence. There tends to be a sense of powerlessness, and many people feel required to cooperate.

Compromise and bargaining.   Another approach to resolving intergroup conflict where agreement is seen as possible involves splitting the difference through compromise, bargaining, or trading. Agreements like these are made even though reservations and unresolved issues which initially separated the groups still remain. "Splitting" mechanisms are used by many negotiators in settling intergroup win/lose struggles. The idea is to convert the conflict into a situation where agreement is possible. Various forms of splitting the difference occur in groups where continued disagreement is more costly than some type of resolution. A good bargain occurs when the leaders find that one group desires something that the other group possesses and vice versa. The conditions are such that an exchange can leave both sides in a higher state of fulfillment than before the bargaining. The arrangement between many groups in organizations involves trading or exchanging favors. One group may agree to take a specific action which carries some loss to itself on the condition that the other group is bound to return the favor at some future time. This describes the characteristic of equal deprivation or equal sacrifice and often is perceived as an essential feature that balances equal gain. Therefore, bargaining is sometimes a pessimistic concept, the acceptable alternative to a win/lose situation. When no one best answer can be worked out a compromise resolution results in something that fits in some respects but fails in others. The individual's or group's point of view makes a difference in that they are accepting the compromise or bargaining position. It is a situation in which neither side wins but neither side loses. If a fair trade is achieved, both sides can feel satisfied.

Mutual problem solving. Mutual intergroup problem solving involves a positive point of view. This approach holds that resolutions are possible between and among groups which are superior to those achieved by working independently, struggling in a win/lose situation, or even by bargaining. A precondition for problem solving is a more optimistic feeling toward the capabilities of the other group. Intergroup problem solving is focused on solving the problem, not accommodating different points of view. It involves identifying the causes of the reservation, doubt, and misunderstanding among the groups and exploring alternative ways of approaching the conflict. The alternative solutions which develop may not be held by either of the groups before they begin working together. When the groups develop alternative resolutions, they are involved in experimental trying of those approaches. The testing provides an indication of the quality of the situation. When groups are truly involved in problem-solving behaviors, the representatives become links between the groups. The achievement of agreements and integration of group efforts are built on the understanding, confidence, trust, and respect for each other.

Problem solving between groups can occur when the groups recognize that the problem is the relationship between the groups rather than difficulties inherent in the groups separately. Therefore, if the problem is in the relationship, solutions involve resolving issues in that relationship and sharing the responsibility for seeing that the solutions work. Success in working together will be seen through the superordinate goals which emerge from their joint effort. The superordinate goals will provide opportunities for broader cooperation. Such opportunities can provide both groups with the attainment of goals not possible through independent interactions.

Blake and colleagues (1964) describe the behaviors necessary for intergroup problem solving. The first step involves a joint definition of the problems. Facts are not explored from separate standpoints but are viewed by and through intergroup contact, with both groups or their representatives sitting together to identify the issues that separate them and the problems that require solution. The advantage of this approach is that the problems separating the two groups are found to be quite different from the problems described individually by the groups.

The second step in this problem-solving method is for a full problem review. This is not done by subcommittees but involves all the members or as many members as possible from both groups. This communicates the fundamental facts and issues to all the members and provides an opportunity for them to present additional facts. This also provides a setting for the final definition of the problem to insure that it is valid.

The next step involves developing a range of alternatives in dealing with each of the identified problems. This stage will involve working through joint subgroups. The membership of these subgroups have an opportunity to present alternatives to each other whose identification might otherwise not have occurred.

The result of these alternatives is again reported to the combined groups, and the larger intergroup has an opportunity to debate the alternatives. This joint reporting provides an opportunity for additional alternatives to be explored.

The searching for possible solutions for each of the alternative issues is the next step. It is not intended to rank the solutions but to test those alternatives which seem realistic and feasible.

Another step in the process involves a combined group evaluating each of the proposed solutions. This permits a test of these solutions and provides an opportunity for combinations of solutions or new solutions to be discovered through the interchange in the large group discussion.

A final step involves the whole intergroup weighing the alternative solutions. This may begin by a subgroup ranking each solution and its advantages and disadvantages and then presenting these ranked solutions to the combined groups for their review and selection. The selection that seems best in terms of the facts and events can then be chosen from the rankings.

The important aspect of these stages is that it is the joint subgroups and joint intergroup meetings that evaluate the possible solutions for the problems that they have identified. If intergroup problem solving can be attained, each group is in a position to retain its autonomy while each is able to make its contribution to the goals they share in common.

Intervention into Intergroup Conflict

The interventions the consultant might use to resolve intergroup conflicts are based primarily on his or her assumptions regarding conflict. If the assumption is that conflict is inevitable and that agreement is impossible, then the method used would involve fate, third-party judgments, or a win/lose strategy. If one's assumption is that conflict is not necessarily inevitable but that agreement is impossible, the methods of neutrality, isolation, or withdrawal are likely to be discussed. When agreement is seen as possible, different interventions may be employed including peaceful coexistence or some type of bargaining. As stated earlier, all of these approaches involve a pessimistic point of view and leave both sides with a certain amount of loss even when things go their way. Mutual problem solving, however, such as third-party consultation, assumes that effective collaborations can be gained and that through joint interactions both sides can retain an appropriate amount of independence while achieving an overall larger success.

Traditional Third-Party Interventions

When individuals or representatives of opposing sides have been unable to reach a reconciliation, third-parties are regarded as a means to bring the two parties together to settle their differences. The traditional third-party approaches to conflict resolution are conciliation, mediation, and arbitration.

Conciliation. Conciliation usually implies a close relationship of the participants to the third-party intervener. It is concerned with activities that help lead participants to an agreement rather than settling differences and allocating values according to past practices. It is an active role rather than one of interpretation and may include efforts to include and clarify facts. Examination of the disagreement may lead to recommendations or formal findings which the participants could be expected to accept. Success or failure depends to some degree on the relationships established between the conciliator and the participants. The role of the conciliator is to pacify and try to insure that the participants do not react against each other but consider their responses (Burton, 1969).

The techniques used in conciliation are directed toward improving personal relations and are seen to be most useful in disputes where the two parties are not committed to representing larger groups and where negotiations are primarily personal and focused on shorter-term consequences. These techniques are more likely to be regarded with suspicion in actual disagreements between employers and unions (Webb, 1986).

Mediation. The third party in mediation uses an influential, substantive role that may employ either a process-oriented method directed at harmonizing relations between the two parties to improve their mutual understanding of the different offers or a content-oriented method directed at discovering a negotiated resolution to the differences (Webb, 1986).

The mediator may present the case of each party to the other when the parties are not willing to meet face to face; however, the third party also serves to mediate between two parties who have come together to present their own perspectives, with the third party there to clarify communication. More difficulties are involved when the parties do not meet face to face because the mediator has to represent the point of view of one party to the other. In such meetings the third party may become identified with the interests of the party he or she is presenting, and, if the mediation continues for a longer period of time, the disputants may have difficulty accepting the third party as a neutral position (Burton, 1969).

Douglas (1962), discussing the stages in mediation, stated that conflict between the two parties was central to the process of mediation rather than just a result of misunderstandings. During the resolution process, mediators need to assist the two parties in differentiating between their stances as party representatives and their need to maintain a viable, personal relationship with their opposites. Resolved disputes tend to progress through three stages: from the establishment of a bargaining range, which emphasizes the extent of their interparty disagreement; to a stage of tentative exploration of possible settlements, where negotiators search for signs of agreement; to a decision-making crisis in which party relationships are again predominant.

Arbitration.　Arbitration is the settlement of a disagreement by the decision of an arbitrator who interprets existing law or rules and binds the participants to a decision. Arbitration can take into account nonlegal arguments, and it may be held in secret. The procedures generally are more flexible than judicial processes though they tend to follow the practices of law in giving and sifting evidence. The participants may be involved in the selection of the arbitrator, which enhances their confidence in the process. Arbitration is only one step away from judicial review; therefore, it has many of the drawbacks of the judicial system and few of the advantages of greater participation by the participants in the decision making (Burton, 1969). Since voluntary settlement is the favored norm of conflicting parties, arbitration is regarded paradoxically as being more successful the less it is used. Comparison of the types of arbitration indicate that the two parties act strategically depending on whether they expect the arbitrator to offer a compromise or choose the final offer of either side (Webb, 1986).

Research.　Rubin's (1980) review of experimental research on third-party interventions included three assertions. First, third parties assist in making concessions without loss of face, providing more rapid and effective conflict resolution. Second, intervention methods which are effective in lower-intensity conflict may be ineffective or even exacerbate the problem when conflict is high. Third, disputing parties in a conflict may see the third-party intervention as unwelcome and an unwanted intrusion. They may wish to solve their conflicts on their own. Holzworth (1983) reported support for Rubin's third assertion. The mediator's efforts in a cognitive conflict model did not seem to be considered necessary by the judges in any condition of that experiment.

McGillicuddy, Welton, and Pruitt (1987) conducted a field experiment to compare three models of third-party intervention: straight mediation, mediation/arbitration (same), and mediation/arbitration (different). The intervention models differed according to what happened if agreements between the disputing parties were not reached. In straight mediation, the hearing ended; in mediation/arbitration (same), the same third party arbitrated; while in the mediation/arbitration (different), a fourth party not present during the mediation hearings arbitrated. Findings indicated that the disputing parties in mediation/arbitration (same) participated in more problem solving and were less competitive and hostile than the disputing parties in straight mediation. The disputing parties in the mediation/arbitration (different) were intermediate on these dimensions. Notable differences in the third party's behavior were found in that mediation/arbitration (different) parties were less involved throughout the session than those in the other two conditions. The authors proposed three possible explanations for this difference in third-party behavior: (1) the mediators in the mediation/arbitration (different) model may have felt less responsible for the case because another person could be relied on to take over the arbitration; (2) the mediators could have become demoralized seeing themselves as low-power individuals in the process that could be dominated by high-power figures at a later time; and (3) the disputing parties could see the mediator as a weak figure in comparison to the arbitrator waiting to make a decision. Although the mediation/arbitration (same) model was more successful in this study, it was applied only to the mediation phase of the hearing. Other problems could be described for this procedure if the hearing was to go to arbitration. One difficulty involves mediators meeting with the disputing parties in private sessions from which the adversary is excluded. Although such sessions are valuable in locating alternatives to which both parties might agree, it denies the adversary an opportunity to hear or refute evidence that could be prejudicial to his case. Should the mediator become an arbitrator, the judgment may be biased by this secret testimony.

Conclusion.   Webb (1986) notes that the three types of intervention are less distinctive in practice. Much of the research in industrial disputes has been directed toward demonstrating the effectiveness of such interventions and producing settlements; however, the results have been mixed. Sheppard (1984) noted that one of the trends in recent work on conflict intervention has been an increased appreciation of the similarity of techniques available to use in diverse settings. A limitation here, however, is the preoccupation with comparing only the procedures utilized in more formal (e.g., industrial relations) or professional (e.g., process consultation) intervention settings rather than others used in less formal circumstances (e.g., managers, parents, teachers, colleagues, clergy).

THIRD-PARTY CONSULTATION

Third-party consultation has many similarities with the traditional methods, yet it is unique. A perspective on third-party consultation can be gained by reviewing a model developed by Fisher (1972, 1976). This model will provide an overview since it is based on the positions of Walton (1969), Bell and associates (1969), and Doob (1970).

The objectives of third-party consultation include improving the attitudes of the two parties regarding each other; improving the relationship from a destructively competitive one to a collaborative, trusting, problem-solving one; and resolving conflict, which involves solutions agreed upon and committed to by the individuals participating in the process.

The role of the consultant requires that a person be a skilled scholar/practitioner with a background enabling one to be impartial toward two disputing parties. The consultant's professional knowledge and expertise should facilitate productive confrontation between the disputants. It is necessary that the consultant have only a moderate knowledge of the two parties, low power over them, but high control over the consulting situation in which they meet. The variables in the identity of the consultant lay the foundation for each participant's trust, respect, and understanding.

The consultant makes arrangements for the social and physical meeting, arranging for one or more informal and flexible discussions which will focus on the nature of the conflict in a neutral setting. The role of the consultant is both facilitative and diagnostic, yet nonevaluative and noncoercive regarding the outcomes. The conduct and control of the meeting process is the primary goal. The consultant's functions primarily involve inducing positive motivation for the participants, improving communication between them, diagnosing the conflict, and regulating the interaction between the participants. The functions of the consultant are operationalized through specific tactics and procedures. These include holding preliminary interviews with the participants and clarifying communication.

When the consultant is successful in carrying out the functions, he or she establishes the process of assessing the variables in the conflict, managing the conflict, and moving toward conflict resolution. The conduct of these activities will assist in reaching the long-term objectives of the third-party consultation.

Interpersonal Peacekeeping

A more detailed analysis of third-party consultation is gained from Walton's interpersonal peacemaking model. Walton (1969) made a major contribution to the theory and practice of third-party consultation by focusing on the consultant helping two people in an organization manage their interpersonal conflict. His model presents a scheme for diagnosing recurring conflicts between people and then uses the understanding of the interpersonal conflicts to establish strategic functions of the third-party consultant to facilitate a constructive confrontation of the conflict. Although the concepts are focused on interpersonal conflicts in organizations, they are certainly more generally applicable. Interpersonal conflict includes interpersonal disagreement over substantive issues that could occur in any workplace or social system and also on interpersonal conflicts that focus more on the personal and emotional differences between two interdependent people.

The innumerable interdependent situations in life make interpersonal conflicts inevitable. A unique contribution of Walton's position is his idea that a consultant must identify the personal and organizational tendencies which limit the direct approaches to conflict. Such inhibiting factors can be used to manage the conflict and surface it at the most appropriate time and under the most appropriate conditions.

Confrontation involves the two individuals engaging each other directly and focusing on the conflict between them. The objectives of such a confrontation include increasing the authenticity of the relationship to allow the principals to experience increased personal integrity, to increase their commitment to improve the relationship, to diagnose the conflict, to increase their sense of control in their relationship, and to discover and experiment with ways to deescalate the conflict.

Cyclical Diagnostic Model

Walton (1969) described a cyclical diagnostic model pertaining to conflicts between two people. Figure 1 indicates that the individuals may occasionally engage in open conflict and at other times the issues will represent a covert conflict. Something occurs that triggers opposition between the people, and they engage in conflict-relevant behaviors. They experience

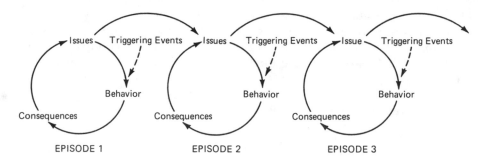

the consequence of this interaction which could lead to resolution. If it does not lead to resolution, the consequence of their interaction will then lead the conflict to become covert again. This type of conflict tends to be dynamic and may escalate or deescalate from one cycle to the next. If people fail to understand the problem and how to resolve it, the conflict may be repeated. The model suggests that to diagnose the situation, the third-party consultant needs to search the issues involved in the problem, the triggering events which set off the conflict, the interpersonal conflict behaviors they exhibit, and the outcomes or consequences of the conflict.

Triggering events.   As seen in the figure, issues that cause problems between two people can and do exist in covert conflict for periods of time. This latent period is maintained by barriers to overt conflict, but circumstances exist which can create an open conflict. Understanding such triggering events and conflict behaviors helps the consultant understand the real issues in a conflict situation.

Numerous behaviors can prevent a person from initiating or reacting to a triggering situation. One person may be inhibited from confronting either the situation or other person due to internal forces. These might be personal attitudes, values, needs, fears, or habitual behaviors; perceptions of others vulnerability; or personal vulnerability. Despite these barriers some events or circumstances can precipitate an open conflict. It is important to understand the types of barriers that are customarily used by each individual and what triggers the open conflict. This level of understanding can be used in several ways to handle the conflict. First, each person can learn to manage the conflict if she or he understands the barriers that she or he and the other individual use as well as what triggers the conflict. The person is then better able to choose the right time and place as well as the appropriate issue for dealing with the conflict. If the preference is to avoid an open conflict, at least temporarily, one can take steps to bolster the barriers and head off the triggering events. In addition, an analysis of the events which surround and precede a conflict may provide cues to primary issues in a recurring conflict. The frequency of the conflict may be controlled by operating on the barriers or triggering events.

Conflict behaviors.   Conflict behaviors involve the tactics used as well as the overtures toward resolution. The conflict tactics may include expressions of feelings such as anger, attack, or avoidance and rejection. The behaviors also include competitive strategies intended to win the conflict such as blocking, interrupting, depreciating the other, forming alliances, and outmaneuvering neutral individuals, criticizing the other person, blaming the other person for the problem, challenging that person's judgment, and forming alliances with someone in a superior position.

Another part of conflict behavior includes the overtures toward a resolution. Such overtures involve cooperative strategies intended to win the conflict such as a search for integrated solutions. Additional behaviors include agreeing to meet, listening to the other side, expressing regret about the difficult, and acknowledging fault.

The consultant's role in this aspect of diagnosing involves helping each person understand his or her own feelings and behaviors when the conflict comes into the open as well as developing an understanding of the other person's feelings and behaviors. This approach to diagnosis contributes to insight into one's self and others and can lead to behavior change.

Consequences.   The consultant and the two parties must examine the consequences of the conflict. They need to be aware of the potential costs and benefits of conflict which affect each person. An appreciation of the magnitude of the costs and benefits is essential for the consultant. Does the risk of improvement justify the risk of trying? An analysis of the particular consequences of a recurrent conflict will provide an understanding of why the conflict is escalating or deescalating.

Issues.   Obviously, the issues are the most important features of the diagnostic model; however, individuals entering into a conflict may not be able to identify the issues or may choose not to specify the real issues. Therefore, the consultant often begins by focusing on the triggering events, which will give some indication of the specific issues. The triggering issues may, in fact, give a clearer indication of the issues than either the conflict behaviors or the consequences.

A clear distinction is made between substantive and emotional issues in a conflict. The substantive issues involve disagreements over policies or rules while emotional issues involve feelings between the individuals. Substantive issues are basically cognitive while the emotional conflicts are affective. The consultants and the two negotiating individuals should not focus on one aspect of the issue while ignoring the other. They may feel comfortable discussing the substantive issue but there needs to be attention to the emotional component as well.

Diagnosing conflicts requires discriminating between issues that are basic and those that are merely symptomatic and represent a proliferation of the primary issues. An individual may inject a second or substantive issue into a conflict because it provides a more socially acceptable issue for the contention. The primary issue could risk so much embarrassment for one or both individuals that they detour to symptomatic issues which only reflect the basic issue. In some cases the eventual resolution of the symptomatic issue may lead to a resolution of the primary issue as well. Once the issues are defined, there is better understanding by the individuals. Substantive conflicts generally require bargaining and problem solving while emotional conflicts require restructuring of individuals' perceptions and then working through the feelings between them.

Third-Party Strategic Functions

We have stated that it is possible to have a conflict resolved by allowing two parties to pursue their own strategies of avoidance, constraint, or coping. The use of a third-party confrontation, therefore, must be considered an optional step in the management of a conflict. Although well-managed confrontations allow for an exchange of information between the people and increases the authenticity of their relationship, it is possible for confrontations to lead to further polarization of the two positions, increase the personal costs of the conflict, or discourage the people from further efforts to resolve their conflict. Clearly a third-party consultation aims to maximize the gains while minimizing the potential risks. The effectiveness of the third-party intervention depends on the key functions the consultant performs (Walton, 1969).

Assess motivation.   It is important for the consultant to assess the motivation of both individuals in reducing the conflict. If mutual desire to enter the process is lacking, the consultant can delay or avoid a direct meeting. If there is some interest by both people but one has higher motivation, the consultant can help that individual to moderate the level of energy invested in the process and pace him or herself accordingly. The third-party consultant both assesses the motivation and works to achieve a level of symmetry of the motivation for the meeting.

Balance power.   Since an imbalance of situational power affects the course of the confrontation by undermining trust or inhibiting dialogue, the consultant attempts to achieve a balance of power. This may be done by involving more allies for one of the persons or regulating the interaction process in a way that assists the individual with the lesser skills. Another major function of the third-party consultant, then, is to achieve some balance in the power.

Synchronize readiness. Another important function of the consultant is to insure that one person's initiative to enter the meeting is synchronized with the other person's readiness. Should one person seek the confrontation and then be refused by the other, there could be heightened feelings of rejection and the conciliatory gesture could be interpreted as a sign of weakness. The theme of symmetry in the consultant's role, therefore, includes synchronizing the readiness of both individuals to enter the meeting.

Differentiation and integration. The actual confrontation meeting involves both a period of differentiation and a period of integration. The consultant should insure that the period of differentiation is worked through before the session moves on to the integrative stage. Actually, it may take more than one phase of differentiation to clearly describe the parties' differences and their points of view and feelings before they are truly ready to move toward some integration. It is also important that each individual not only states a position during the differentiation but also receives some indication that these views and feelings are understood by the other person. An effective meeting involves an integration in which the individuals understand their similarities, acknowledge their common objectives, own up to the positive aspects of their ambivalences, and engage in positive actions to manage their conflict. A successful third-party consultant will need to be comfortable with a high level of division and hostility during the differentiation phase as well as during the warmth and closeness that may be expressed during the integration phase.

Assess openness. The consultant assesses the factors that contribute to openness in dialogue. These may include organizational norms regarding the expression of differences, the emotional reassurances to the individual, and the skills for facilitating the discussion. It is helpful when the consultant can affect the norms for this discussion and be perceived as a source of emotional support for the process.

Reliability of communication. Contributing to the reliability of the interpersonal communication is a major function of the consultant. The consultant may need to translate or restate messages until both the sender and receiver agree on the meaning. Another aspect of the reliability of communications is the development of a common language regarding the substantive issues, emotional issues, and the meeting process itself.

Optimum tension.   The consultant can attempt to achieve an optimum level of tension during the meeting. At times he or she may raise the tension level in order to create a sense of urgency or to increase the amount and importance of the information exchanged. At other times he or she might wish to relax the level of threat when it begins to produce rigidity in one or both of the parties or is possibly producing defensiveness in their communication.

Walton concludes that none of these functions are sufficient alone. All are necessary for a successful third-party confrontation. Although he hypothesizes that each function is capable of influencing the improvement or resolution of the conflict, the other aspects should be present in adequate amounts. The more symmetrical the situational power of the people, the more successful will be the confrontation meeting.

Third-Party Tactics

A discussion of tactics describes the practice of a third-party consultant. Certainly the third-party consultant's functions and tactics are interrelated. The tactics are the behaviors which the consultant uses in performing the functions. There are five major areas for third-party interventions: the presence of the consultant, preliminary interviewing, structuring the context of the meeting, intervening in the process, and assisting in the follow-up.

Presence.   The least active intervention of a consultant is being available and present in the meeting. Often just the presence of a third party in a situation performs a synchronizing function. The presence of another person also influences norms related to openness and can assure the individuals who see him/her as a source of emotional support. The consultant's presumed possession of skills also decreases the sense of risking failure and can facilitate dialogue.

Preliminary interviewing.   It is important for the consultant to have a preliminary interview with each of the individuals prior to the confrontation meeting. These meetings are used to assess the motivation of each individual and obtain other relevant information about his or her substantive and emotional issues. It also provides an opportunity to assess the openness of each individual and to provide better basis for deciding whether to proceed with the confrontation meeting. Knowledge of both individuals and their perspectives puts the third-party consultant in a position to be more skillful in managing the dialogue with the two individuals.

Structuring the meeting.   Structuring the context of the meeting is an important tactic for the consultant. He or she can influence the physical and social atmosphere by choosing a neutral site and one that provides symmetry in terms of the situational power of the participants. The degree of formality can be established by the method of seating, the formality of addressing each individual, and the degree of urgency versus relaxation in the interaction. It is important that an open-ended time period is scheduled and that the confrontation meeting is not interrupted. The consultant controls many factors in the meeting by determining the composition of the meeting. Including other persons in the meeting can increase the relevant perceptions and insights, the available support for one or both individuals, the perceived risk for one or both persons, and the importance of the larger organizational reality in which the people must ultimately work.

Intervene in discussion. Consultants can intervene directly in the discussion throughout the process. They may initiate the agenda for the meeting, thereby providing the focus of the discussion. By providing equal airtime, they are able to control part of the power in the situation. Terminating a repetitive discussion, rewording constructive behaviors, and punishing destructive behaviors are included as referee-oriented tactics. In terms of communication, consultants restate, summarize, translate, and encourage feedback to the participants. Consultants also may give feedback and offer diagnostic insights. They may offer techniques that will assist the individuals in joining issues and engaging each other in the process.

Follow-up. Some third-party consultations resolve the conflict in one meeting; however, many involve more than one meeting. Consultants need to assist the individuals in planning and preparing for further dialogue, whether in a third-party meeting or in continued individual interactions. It is important that they have helped the participants understand the ingredients that make a dialogue productive and identify for them the techniques and principles that were used effectively in this particular meeting. Through this part of the work consultants increase their ability to continue the dialogue on their own. It may be important for them to provide continuing third-party participation in further meetings. If that is apparent at the close of the first meeting, they should follow up and establish another meeting time.

Third-party consultant attributes. There are five role attributes for the third-party consultant using this type of conflict intervention: (1) high professional expertise in social processes, (2) low power over the fate of the participants, (3) high control over the confrontation meeting, (4) moderate knowledge about the individuals' issues and background information, and (5) neutrality with respect to the substantive outcome as well as personal relationships.

INTERVENTION STRATEGIES

Intervention strategies used in social conflict within organizations are generally treated in the literature in a rather isolated way. They are seldom compared with other possible strategies and then not as part of a more comprehensive framework. Prein (1987) studied the extent to which some of the main strategies described in the literature are applied by internal and external organizational consultants. From his review the approaches most often used by organizational consultants involved mediation and consultation. The review of the literature identified five methods of third-party influence.

Focusing on the Process

The consultant can try to enhance direct contact and confrontation between the two parties by focusing on the communication process between them, helping them to formulate their points of view, express their feelings and emotions, raise underlying personal matters, and listen better to each other. The consultant can also provide procedures for better communication by participants or try to improve their skills, but can also contribute to the process by giving observations, expressing understanding, showing support and acceptance, and by providing information about interaction in communication processes.

Focus on Procedures

A consultant may regulate the interaction between the two parties by setting up and observing interaction rules. The consultant could define conflict management as a negotiation process and then provide procedures for that process, or he or she could define it as a decision-making process and provide methods for problem identification and decision making.

Focus on the Content

The consultant may intervene more directly in the content of the conflict by being involved personally in fact finding. He or she may divide the issues into smaller and more manageable ones or may even attempt a convergence of both points of view by giving more information to each party about the position and viewpoints of the other or by making suggestions for possible situations.

Influencing Behavior

A third party may have influence due to his or her own personal characteristics or by using external pressure from superiors for public opinion. A third party could have power on the basis of the contact between him or herself and the two parties or because the parties consider him or her as competent, objective, credible, and impartial. The third party may have a reputation as an expert in relations, in content issues, and serve as a model. The consultant may have power as a result of external support as well as a good social reputation.

Goals

The third party may work to achieve various goals. One type of goal would be to find a fully acceptable solution to both parties in the conflict issue. This would improve the relationship, prevent repetition, and teach the participants to manage their future conflicts more adequately. Other types of goals would include creating a clearer, more workable situation in which to find a pragmatic solution and learn from the conflict without necessarily resolving it. Another approach would be to work on more structural solutions by altering the organization of work and establishing better rules and procedures.

Empirically Based Classification of Strategies

Prein (1987) conducted a study to discover the extent to which primary strategies, extrapolated from the literature, were used by internal and external organizational consultants in their practice. The concept of conflict used in the study included incompatible interests/goals/values/views, as well as more subjective, psychological consequences and the reactions of the two parties. Prein used both a Likert-scale questionnaire and interview data with practicing third-party consultants who presented 69 cases of third-party intervention. The analysis revealed four clusters of strategies similar to those identified in the literature. Two major strategies, consultation and mediation, were found. Consultation was divided into two types of strategies that had a process approach in common but differed in that one focused on confrontation and the other on a procedural approach.

The first cluster yields a consultation strategy emphasizing direct confrontation of the underlying points of difference and expressions of emotion with a purpose to become completely free, achieve greater clarity, and improve mutual relations. This was identified as the confrontation approach. The analysis of the interviews with the third-party consultants adds clarity to the findings of the cluster analysis. The third-party consultants in the first cluster attached more importance to the responsibility and self-involvement of the two disputants; therefore, their readiness to work together on a solution was considered crucial. The consultant's primary orientation is toward confrontation on the points of difference; therefore, these consultants did not conduct individual interviews with the involved participants beforehand. They aimed to give the two parties an opportunity to talk to each other and create an atmosphere in which they could feel safe in speaking without it being reported to superiors in the organization. In successful cases, after one or two sessions of confronting the issues, a breakthrough may be achieved and a third party may become less involved. In unsuccessful cases, however, the problems may emerge around the point of direct confrontation; participants will not want to continue and may dismiss the third party. Evaluation of the results of this type of consultation typically involves improvement of climate, atmosphere, and mutual cooperation.

The second cluster shows a process-oriented way of working with more emphasis on procedures for both identifying problems and decision-making. The third party uses more personal influence but not pressure tactics. He or she is oriented both toward improving mutual relationships and looking for structural, stable solutions for the specific problem. This was identified as a procedural approach. In the analysis of procedural-style interviews, there is less emphasis on confrontation and more on problem solving. The third-party role involves creating and implementing solutions, often by giving directions to the process. The disputing parties are left almost completely free to choose in that the third party uses no pressure tactics to get them to agree to his or her proposals. The results of this strategy are evaluated in terms of the good solution, improved working atmosphere, and mutual relationships.

The third cluster reveals a strategy in which the third party focuses on the content of the conflict and places pressure on the participants. This cluster is not particularly concerned with improving mutual relations but focuses on seeing that the situation will be workable and finding a pragmatic compromise for the specific problem. This strategy was labeled mediation.

According to the interview analysis, in the mediation strategy of the third cluster, it seems necessary that the third party be invited by the two disputing parties. Since the third party's function is in the substantive area, he or she can give the impression of seeming to take sides. This third-party strategy sometimes uses the consultant's relationships with superiors to implement certain solutions. The third party generally interviews the two participants individually, which insures that he or she will be informed and therefore can either influence or pressure the parties to accept suggestions. The results of this strategy are manifested in terms of achieving an often unavoidable compromise solution.

The fourth cluster identifies a strategy in which the third party attempts very little. It appears this party had none of the power available to the third parties in the other groups of cases. This approach was labeled a powerless or unsure third party. The interview analysis suggests that in the powerless or unsure third-party strategy, the individual may have been asked in for something entirely different than this conflict. This person appears to work reluctantly and may not believe in his or her position. The consultant may try to avoid confrontation between the parties, not feeling competent for this work and expecting resistance from the two participants. Consultants with this strategy take a distant position and appear reluctant to react, keeping themselves in the background and letting things happen. Actually, this approach is not a strategy but more of a nonstrategy.

A Contingency Approach

Prein (1984) proposed a contingency approach which assumed that there is no one best way of intervening in all types of conflicts but that the intervention strategy chosen should depend on the type of conflict and the context in which it occurs. The contingency model included three elements: (1) a topology of intervention strategies, (2) the problem to be changed and the context in which it occurs, and (3) the effectiveness of different strategies. He used the topology of strategies described from the literature as well as reported in his cluster analysis. One of these approaches was the confrontation consulting strategy which emphasized the direct confrontation of underlying points of disagreement and expression of emotions aimed at creating clarity and improving mutual relations. The second strategy was the procedural approach, which emphasizes the process-oriented method of working with emphasis on the procedures for identifying problems and decision making. The third strategy, titled mediation, involved the consultant focusing on the content of the conflict and using pressure with the two parties to find a workable compromise for the specific problem.

Prein (1984) concluded that the strategy of confrontation would be most applicable for conflicts that have not escalated and are not too complicated, being primarily founded on communication differences, misunderstandings, distrust, and irritations. Both disputing parties must be motivated to work on their conflicts. The presence of some norms and rules of openness and fair play seem to have a positive effect on the results of the confrontation strategy.

The strategy of the procedural approach is much stronger than the other two and has a very broad application area. This strategy can be effectively applied to conflicts that have already escalated and that are somewhat complicated. With the communication and emotional disturbances of a conflict, a process approach which uses more direction is appropriate. The third party needs room to maneuver so that the two disputing parties have some flexibility, no standard solution is apparent, and there is no interference from external spectators. As in most consultation, the two parties must have an appropriate level of motivation to solve the problems themselves.

The mediation strategy was reported to be more appropriate for conflicts that have not escalated and that have yet to become deadlocked. Mediation is also appropriate for problems that deal with substantive issues such as material interests, roles, and job content.

SUMMARY

In discussing the concept of conflict behavior, this chapter examined the assumptions the disputing parties may have. Their assumptions about whether conflict is inevitable and whether agreement is possible affect the behaviors of the disputing parties and impact on the consultant's role. Three traditional approaches to conflict resolution were reviewed. Those set the stage for presenting third-party consultation, which focuses on diagnosing and helping the disputing parties to resolve their conflict by emphasizing the importance of communication and relationship between the two parties. A diagnostic model presented in the chapter helps consultants understand the problems between such individuals. The model also examines the functions and tactics of the consultant. The chapter concludes with some research on the third-party consultation intervention strategies.

REFERENCES

BELL, R., CLEVELAND, S., HANSON, P., and O'CONNELL, W. (1969). Small group dialogue and discussion: An approach to police–community relationships. *Journal of Criminal Law, Criminology and Police Science*, 3, 242–246.

BLAKE, R. R., SHEPHARD, H. A., and MOUTON, J. S. (1964). *Managing intergroup conflict in industry*. Houston: Gulf Publishing Company.

BURTON, J. (1969). *Conflict and communication: The use of controlled communication in internation relations*. London: McMillan.

DOOB, L. (ed.) (1970). *Resolving conflict in Africa: The Fermeda Workshop*. New Haven, CT: Yale University Press.

DOUGLAS, A. (1962). *Industrial peacemaking*. New York: Columbia University Press.

FISHER, R. (1972). Third-party consultation: A method for the study and resolution of conflict. *Journal of Conflict Resolution*, 16, 67–94.

FISHER, R. (1976). Third-party consultation: A skill for professional psychologists in community practice. *Professional Psychology*, 12, 344–351.

HOSZWORTH, J. (1983). Intervention in a cognitive conflict. *Organizational Behavior in Human Performance*, 32, 216–231.

McGILLICUDDY, N., WELTON, G., and PRUITT, D. (1987). Third-party intervention: A field experiment pairing three different models. *Journal of Personality and Social Psychology*, 53, 104–112.

PREIN, H. (1987). Strategies for third-party intervention. *Human Relations*, 40, 699–720.

PREIN, H. (1984). A contingency approach for conflict intervention. *Group and Organizational Studies*, 9, 81–102.

RUBIN, J. (1980). Experimental research on third-party intervention in conflict: Toward some generalizations. *Psychological Bulletin*, 87, 379–391.

SHEPPARD, B. (1984). Third-party conflict intervention: A procedural framework. In B. Staw and L. Cummings (eds.), *Research in organizational behavior*. Greenwich, CT: JAI Press.

WALTON, R. (1969). *Interpersonal peacemaking, confrontations, and third-party consultation*. Reading, MA: Addison-Wesley.

WEBB, J. (1986). Third-parties at work: Conflict resolution or social control? *Journal of Occupational Psychology*, 59, 247–258.

INDEX